ST. JOHN'S

NATURE'S REMEDIES

ST. JOHN'S WORT

The Natural Anti-depressant and More

Andrew Chevallier, FNIMH

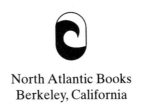

North Atlantic Books
Berkeley, California

First published 1999 by Souvenir Press Ltd., 43 Great Russell Street, London, WC1B 3PA

This edition published by
North Atlantic Books
P.O. Box 12327
Berkeley, California 94712

Cover redesign by Catherine Campaigne
Text typeset by Rowland Phototypesetting Ltd., Bury St. Edmunds, Suffolk

St. John's Wort: The Natural Anti-depressant, and More is sponsored by the Society for the Study of Native Arts and Sciences, a nonprofit educational corporation whose goals are to develop an educational and crosscultural perspective linking various scientific, social, and artistic fields; to nurture a holistic view of arts, sciences, humanities, and healing; and to publish and distribute literature on the relationship of mind, body, and nature.

Library of Congress Cataloging-in-Publication Data

ISBN 1-55643-331-X

1 2 3 4 5 6 7 8 9 / 03 02 01 00 99

To Maria Mercedes

Acknowledgements

Many people have helped in the writing of this book—some unknowingly, like my patients, who invariably teach me far more than they ever realise, and some knowingly:

Carol Symonds, MNIMH, whose determination and enthusiasm in researching the book with me have been invaluable; my colleagues at Middlesex University, especially Celia Bell, Kofi Busia and Ellis Snitcher, whose support and advice have helped me to build the confidence to take on a project such as this; and many fellow medical herbalists, who sustain the view that plant medicines cannot simply be reduced to their constituent parts. And finally Maria, my partner, who has known most about this book by my absence writing it. My thanks and appreciation to all—I would have struggled without them, though all mistakes or omissions are mine.

Andrew Chevallier

Note to Readers

The aim of this book is to provide information on the uses of hypericum in the treatment of relevant diseases. Although every care has been taken to ensure that the advice is accurate and practical, it is not intended to be a guide to self-diagnosis and self-treatment. Where health is concerned—and in particular a serious problem of any kind—it must be stressed that there is no substitute for seeking advice from a qualified medical or herbal practitioner. All persistent symptoms, of whatever nature, may have underlying causes that need, and should not be treated without, professional elucidation and evaluation.

It is therefore very important, if you are considering trying hypericum, to consult your practitioner first, and if you are already taking any prescribed medication, do not stop it.

The Publisher makes no representation, express or implied, with regard to the accuracy of the information contained in this book, and legal responsibility or liability cannot be accepted by the Author or the Publisher for any errors or omissions that may be made or for any loss, damage, injury or problems suffered or in any way arising from following the advice offered in these pages.

Contents

CHAPTER 1

Hypericum—a Modern Medicine?

Used as a medicine since the time of Hippocrates in ancient Greece, hypericum's story is a compelling one, almost a fairy tale. Rejected by nineteenth-century medical scientists as worthless, St John's wort, or *Hypericum perforatum* to give it its full name, has recently become a star. 'Humble wort makes good,' the headlines might say, and with good reason. A scientifically proven treatment for mild to moderate depression and the sense of worthlessness and loss of hope that goes with it, hypericum also looks set to have distinct value in the treatment of viral conditions such as HIV and AIDS and hepatitis C. It has real potential as an anti-cancer treatment, and is an effective wound and tissue healer.

As awareness of the risks attached to taking synthetic medicines has grown, attention has begun to focus on the ability of medicinal plants to provide treatment that is both effective and safe. Modern medicine has become 'complex, effective and potentially dangerous',[1] to quote the Dean of Guy's Hospital Medical School, London, and the dilemma for doctors and patients alike is to find a way through to effective treatment that minimises potential risks. Although it is not yet generally recognised, several medicinal plants have been shown to tread this path successfully, finding a 'middle way' in which clear-cut efficacy is not achieved at the cost of a high incidence of side-effects.

Hypericum is perhaps the prime example of this group of herbs, which includes medicines such as garlic (*Allium sativum*) and ginkgo (*Ginkgo biloba*). In hypericum's case its safety record is remarkable—in 15 clinical studies, involving more than 1,000 patients suffering from depressive illness, those taking a placebo recorded a higher percentage of side-effects (4.8 per cent) than those taking hypericum (4.1 per cent).[2] Hypericum can, of course, cause side-effects and is not suitable for everyone, but in the world of anti-depressants its safety record is second to none.

The resurgence of interest in herbal medicines that has swept hypericum into the headlines reflects a new willingness in people to try out such remedies. Revivals of plant-based medicines have occurred before in the last 150 years. A key difference this time round is the quantity and quality of scientific evidence behind their use, and the increasingly sophisticated processes used in the manufacture of herbal preparations. Mirroring these changes, sales of herbal medicines around the world have grown at a staggering rate during the last ten years—well over 12 per cent a year between 1993 and 1995, and faster since then.[3]

In the USA, expenditure on complementary medicine was $15 billion in the mid-1990s, while in Australia people are thought to spend twice as much on complementary as they do on conventional medicine.[4] Moreover, some economists now consider complementary medicine as a whole to be the fastest growing sector of western economies after microelectronics. Herbal medicine represents a sizeable part of this sector, and today, everywhere you turn there are advertisements for herbal preparations, especially hypericum, with news items, newspaper articles, phone-ins, and hundreds of Internet sites—hypericum, the natural anti-depressant, has rapidly become something of a *cause celebre*!

Much as hypericum's anti-depressant activity lies at the heart of its value as a medicine, herbal practitioners or phytotherapists have always seen it as having a wider use. Regarded as a 'nervine'—having a restorative and tonic action on nervous tissues as a whole—it is useful in a wide variety of conditions affecting the nervous system, especially stress-related problems, nervous exhaustion and depleted emotional states. Other conditions as diverse as burns, stomach ulcers, shingles, toothache and bedwetting will also benefit.

The turning-point in hypericum's fortunes came in 1984 when the German Department of Health published a monograph[5] on St John's wort, listing its medicinal uses. These included 'psycho-somatic disorders, depressive states, anxiety and/or nervous rest-lessness'. Clinical research into the herb had begun in the late 1970s, with the first study[6] indicating that here was a potentially effective anti-depressant with a very low level of side-effects. A huge volume of research, mostly within Germany, has built up on the herb since this time.

Making sense of this research, and explaining its findings, form an important part of this book. Chapters 3 to 5 aim to do just this, focusing on the many different and subtle effects that hypericum has on the human mind and body. However, it is equally a practical book for those wanting to take the herb as a medicine. Chapter 8 gives full details of when hypericum should prove effective and how best to take it—including preparation of infusions, tinctures and oil, and important safety issues. Chapter 2 provides a botanical overview of the plant, with brief instructions for growing, harvesting and storing. Useful addresses and Internet sites are listed as an appendix. Hypericum's uses throughout history—medicinal, folkloric and magical—are looked at in chapter 6. The plant's use in twentieth-century herbal medicine is summarised in chapter 7, which also provides details on using hypericum in combination with a number of key herbal medicines. Chapter 9 examines the herb's future potential in the twenty-first century, and the book concludes with a brief appraisal of its role as a medicine.

HYPERICUM IN MEDICINE

In Germany, well over twenty million people have taken hypericum long term for depressive illness. Almost all GPs prescribe it, it outsells all other anti-depressants, and it is the first, and preferred, treatment for many emotional or affective disorders. The range of other conditions for which it is prescribed includes HIV and AIDS, stomach ulcers, attention deficit disorder (hyperactivity in children) and menopausal problems. Hypericum has what can only be described as an astonishing variety of medical applications.

In the English-speaking world the tide is turning towards natural anti-depressants such as hypericum, although most doctors continue to prescribe anti-depressants such as the 'tricyclic' amitryptiline or 'selective serotonin reuptake inhibitors' like fluoxetine (Prozac) for depressive illness. These synthetic medicines can and do prove effective, though the most often cited reason for discontinuing treatment is the unpleasant side-effects produced. While Prozac has been regarded as a 'wonder drug' of the nineties, it has at the same time inspired a spate of lawsuits from people alleged to have had bad experiences with it.[7] Prozac remains controversial and there are some doctors who are concerned about its potential to cause addiction.

Hypericum is not yet anything like as well researched as Prozac, though medical researchers who have spent time investigating its role as an anti-depressant recognise the therapeutic value of the herb. Here is the view of one of the leading US researchers on hypericum:

> St John's wort is a remarkably safe anti-depressant with an apparently unique mode of action. Although it has demonstrated efficacy in mild to moderate depression when compared with placebo and tricyclic anti-depressants, several research areas beg to be explored. Its effects should be compared to serotonin reuptake inhibitors (SSRIs).[8]

While the American medical world is beginning to change rapidly in its view of herbal medicines, it seems that in Britain a far more conservative attitude prevails. As one experienced British pharmacognosist, Dr Peter Houghton, noted in a letter to the *British Medical Journal* in 1996, there is 'a need for more clinicians in Britain to be willing to participate in clinical trials of well authenticated herbal medicines'.[9]

Some months after a glowing report on St John's wort in the 5

May 1997 issue of *Newsweek*, in which a hypericum user was quoted as saying, 'I feel restored, I feel my normal self again', details were announced of the largest research project into a herbal medicine ever undertaken. The US Office of Alternative Medicine and National Institute of Mental Health[10] were jointly providing $4.3 million for a three-year, 336-patient study coordinated by the Duke University Medical Center in North Carolina. Hypericum's efficacy as an anti-depressant would be compared with both a synthetic SSRI anti-depressant and a placebo. If the outcome proves positive hypericum will be on the verge of full acceptance as an anti-depressant in the USA.

Hypericum—the 'whole'
Hypericum is a native European wild plant, growing to about 60cm (2ft) in height and bursting into flower towards the end of June. The upper leaves, buds, yellow flowers and seed capsules have the greatest medicinal activity and are gathered on a dry sunny morning. These parts—the 'herb'—are then dried or processed to produce a range of different preparations, typically infusions, tinctures and standardised extracts, which are then taken as medicines. Hypericum can also be prepared as an oil which makes a useful home remedy for minor burns, scalds and wounds.

Throughout history the plant has been associated with the sun and sunlight, often being harvested at around the solstice when hypericum was thought to have greatest power. Even today there is an unexpected link between the plant and the sun—as if it somehow manages to magically store the warmth, light and energy of the midsummer sun in its flowers—and a recurring theme of this book will be how both hypericum and sunlight act in similar ways, helping to relieve depressive 'gloomy' states and the 'winter blues'. Moreover, sunlight dramatically strengthens the antiviral activity of the herb, for example against HIV infection; while too much of the herb (in particular, hypericin) causes photosensitisation and, on exposure to light, burning of the skin in fair-skinned people. In addition, hypericum has been found to contain appreciable levels of melatonin, a hormone intimately connected with the body's natural, circadian rhythms. Produced by the pineal gland at the base of the brain, melatonin is released in response to reduced levels of sunlight, as the days draw in towards winter.

One purpose of dwelling briefly on hypericum and sunlight is to stress the point that it is a natural rather than a human-made medicine. It does not come out of a laboratory but out of the earth, having evolved over millions of years on our planet. As a result, if it is assessed in exactly the same way as a synthetic laboratory-produced medicine, then understanding of the herb will be distorted and material of therapeutic relevance missed. Some important factors affecting herbal medicines are:

- *Natural variability*
  Identical plants grown in different sites, or the same plant in different years, can have significantly different levels of key active constituents.

- *Growing and harvesting methods*
  Artificial fertilisers, herbicides, fungicides and so on may alter the plant's chemical composition and leave harmful residues; time of harvesting and method of drying also influence the quality of the herb.

- *Nutritional value*
  In common with all plants, hypericum contains trace elements; also carbohydrates and seeds rich in polyunsaturated fatty acids.

- *Synergistic activity*
  The many constituents within the plant—both active and inert—collectively produce a greater medicinal effect within the body, for example as an anti-depressant, than constituents given on their own.

The fact that animals and humans have evolved alongside plants, and depend on them for food, is a key reason why medicinal plants, when properly used, have such a low incidence of side-effects. Unlike many synthetic chemical anti-depressants, hypericum does not interact with alcohol, cause addiction, dependence, sexual dysfunction, headaches or impair memory. In fact, it can be used to treat several of these problems, clinical studies indicating that the herb may be of value in the treatment of addictions and headaches.

Hypericum—the 'parts'

Understanding how medicinal plants work as medicines is not an easy task. Almost all contain a variety of active constituents and it may take years of patient laboratory work to begin to tease out and separate them—'breaking down' the plant into its key constituent components. Even then, establishing the chemical identity of each different molecule takes time, while assessing their pharmacological or medicinal activity within the human body is a long-term project, to say the least.

Hypericum has by now become one of the most extensively researched of all medicinal plants, yet only part of its chemical nature and of its range of activity as a medicine is properly understood. Furthermore, plant medicines are complex, natural substances which cannot always be predicted to work in a particular way simply because they contain specific active constituents. Turkey rhubarb (*Rheum palmatum*), for example, works at a low dosage to prevent diarrhoea, while at high dosage it is a powerful laxative. It contains strongly laxative constituents—anthraquinones—but at a low dose their activity is secondary to the binding action of the tannins also present within the root of the plant.[11]

Therefore—and this is the important point—analysing the active constituents of a plant provides much useful data but it does not tell one exactly how the plant works in practice as a 'whole'. In short, the 'parts' give a good idea of how the 'whole' may work but are not the complete explanation.

With this in mind, the following section looks at hypericum and its key constituents, as they are currently understood.

Key constituents of hypericum and their medicinal activity[12, 13]

CONSTITUENT	ACTIVITY	CONCENTRATION
Polycyclic diones[14]	antiviral, anti-inflammatory,	buds, flowers
Hypericin	potential anti-cancer agent	−0.1 – 0.15% in total
Pseudohypericin		
Phloroglucinols[15, 16]	antibacterial, anti-depressant	flowers, fruits
Hyperforin	—inhibits serotonin uptake,	2 – 5% (in fruits)
Adhyperforin	wound healing	0.2 – 2% (in fruits)
Flavonoids	spasmolytic, MAO inhibition,	aerial parts, buds, flowers
Quercetin	antiviral, vasodilator	−2 – 4% in total
Hyperoside		
Rutin		
+ many others		
Proanthocyanidins[17]	antimicrobial, antiviral, vasodilator,	aerial parts, buds, flowers
Catechin	antioxidant, astringent	−6.2 – 12.1% in total
Epicatechin		
Procyanidins		
Biflavones[18]		buds, flowers
Amentoflavone	anti-inflammatory, anti-ulcer,	−0.01 – 0.5% in total
118-biapigenin	sedative	

Hypericum also contains:

Phenylpropanes		
Chlorogenic acid		below 1%
Caffeic acid		very low levels
+ many others		
Xanthones		
Kielcorin		approx. 0.01% in roots
1,3,6,7-tetrahydroxy-xanthone		trace in aerial parts

CONSTITUENT	CONCENTRATION
Essential oil	0.1 – 1.0%; buds, flowers
—2, methyloctane	16.4% of essential oil
—α-pinene	10.6% of essential oil
—β-pinene	
—sesquiteperpenes	
Amino acid derivatives	
Gamma-aminobutyric acid (GABA)	0.7 mg/g
Melatonin[19]	4.39 mcg/g in flowers; 1.75 mcg/g in leaves
Fixed oil[20]	seeds
Linoleic acid	50% of fixed oil
Linolenic acid	31.5% of fixed oil

Key active constituents

Hypericin and pseudohypericin
Of all the constituents within hypericum, the polycyclic diones, hypericin and pseudohypericin, have received most attention. Little wonder really, as hypericin in particular has a pronounced antiviral activity, both protecting uninfected cells from infection and blocking viral replication in infected cells. It has a unique molecular structure, first identified in 1953,[21] in which one-half of the molecule is hydrophilic (water-loving) while the other half is hydrophobic (water-repelling), and it is likely that it bonds to the outer surface of cell membranes.[22] In the presence of light hypericin reacts to release 'singlet oxygen', a powerful oxidant which is probably responsible for the molecule's viricidal activity.[14] Hypericin is currently being researched for its antiviral, anti-cancer and anti-inflammatory activities. It is more or less unique to *Hypericum* species.

Pseudohypericin is structurally similar to hypericin, only differing in the substitution of -OH for -H at C3. Though a small change, this introduction of -OH into the molecule means that it will have an action distinct from hypericin. Pseudohypericin occurs in the plant at about 2–4 times the level of hypericin.[12] Both

Hypericin

Pseudohypericin

molecules are concentrated most in the flowers, are strongly red in colour and are thought to be biogenetically derived from emodin anthrone.

In 1984 the German Kommision E monograph on St John's wort[5] identified hypericin as having a direct anti-depressant activity. It has since been shown to have almost no anti-depressant effects. 'Standardisation of hypericum extracts on hypericin content may therefore offer no guarantee of pharmacological equivalence'.[23]

R = H: Hyperforin
R = CH3: Adhyperforin

Hyperforin and adhyperforin

Hyperforin, a phenolic-like epicatechin, was first identified in 1971 as an antibacterial principle—it has a broad spectrum of antimicrobial activity. Its chemical configuration was not finally established until 1983.[15] Hyperforin occurs in the plant at levels 2.5–10 times greater than adhyperforin;[12] both molecules are relatively unstable, and if the herb is poorly dried will quickly degrade. One of its degradation products, methyl-buten-2-ol, is found in the essential oil and has a sedative action.

Hyperforin was shown to have a strong anti-depressant action only in 1998. It influences levels of many neurotransmitters—serotonin, noradrenaline, dopamine and GABA, and reduces levels of some receptor sites.[16]

Flavonoids

Many different flavonoids occur in hypericum, some having antispasmodic activity, while others in laboratory tests have a marked anti-depressant effect. However, the flavonols responsible for this anti-depressant activity, in particular quercetin, hyperoside and rutin, occur at very low levels within the plant.[12] They have a positive effect on the circulation, especially on the capillaries, similar to though less strong than that of the proanthocyanidins (see below); and contribute to the herb's value as a wound healer. The flavonoids also contribute to the plant's overall antiviral activity.

R = H	Quercetin
R = a-L-rhamnosyl	Quercitrin
R = ß-D-glucosyl	Isoquercitrin
R = ß-D-galactosyl	Hyperoside
R = ß-rutinosyl	Rutin

21

Procyanidin B2

Proanthocyanidins

Representing up to as much as 15 per cent of the dried herb,[12] these constituents are condensed tannins (catechol tannins) with strongly astringent, cicatrising (tightening up tissue), antimicrobial and antiviral activity. Together these actions contribute powerfully to the herb's wound-healing activity. The proanthocyanidins are also classified as flavonoids and are largely responsible for the positive effects hypericum has on the heart and circulation, effects which include relaxation of arteries, improved heart function[17] and improved perfusion through the capillaries. The proanthocyanidins are also strongly antioxidant.

Biflavones

In laboratory experiments, amentoflavone has been found to bind to benzodiazepine receptors[18] and may therefore have sedative properties. However, it is not yet clear whether this happens within

Amentoflavone
13',II8-Biapigenin

22

the body, as the molecule may not cross the blood-brain barrier.[12] It was also found to be partly responsible for the deep red colour of hypericum oil.[21] Both constituents have anti-inflammatory activity and contribute to the herb's value in treating ulcers.

CHAPTER 2

Green Medicine

The best plants stand near other good plants or among them—and the
longer the better, the more with flowers the better, and at the time when
flowers are at their highest.

Paracelsus (1493–1541)

A common wayside plant in many temperate regions, St John's
wort can be found growing in meadows and pastures, on banks,
beside roads and beneath walls—almost always on the sunny rather
than the shady side. In some parts of the world it grows so plenti-
fully that it overruns everything else. There are an estimated
350,000 hectares (1,350 square miles) of St John's wort in Victoria
and New South Wales (in Australia),[1] and in parts of the north-west
of North America it is equally prolific. In England it can occasion-
ally be found growing in great numbers, for example, in fields and
sheltered hillsides on the North Downs.

Botanical description

St John's wort (*Hypericum perforatum* L.) is an erect, many-
stemmed herbaceous perennial commonly about 60cm (2 feet) in
height but sometimes reaching up to 1 metre (3 feet), and usually
flowering from its second year of growth.

Leaves	1.5 to 4cm (½ to 1½in) in length, oval to linear, opposite, sessile, glabrous with translucent glands.
Inflorescence	Branched compound cymes with 25–100 flowers, flat-topped or rounded.
Flowers	5 petals (about 10mm (½in) long), bright yellow

	with black glands on margins only; 5 sepals (5mm (¼in) long) acute, +/– black glands; many stamens (up to 100) in 3–5 clusters; ovary superior, 3 styles.
Fruit	up to 8mm (⅜in) long, brown; with strongly pitted brown seeds.
Stem	two raised lines down stem.[2, 3]

The parts used in medicine are the flowering tops, flowers and seed capsules, with the active constituents being found at higher and higher levels the farther up the plant one goes. The hypericin content is lowest in the stem (0.0004 per cent), and highest in the flowers (2.15 per cent).[1] Hyperforin occurs almost exclusively in the flowers, capsules and seeds, and is highest after flowering— 'flowers contain approx. 2 per cent hyperforin and 0.2 per cent adhyperforin, whereas in the fruits up to 5 per cent hyperforin and 2 per cent adhyperforin are found'.[4]

There are roughly 370 species[2] of the genus *Hypericum* throughout the world, and around 15 in north-western Europe,[3] many of which are quite similar in appearance. The *Hypericum* genus is a member of the Clusiaceae family.

St John's wort in the wild

Except in high alpine regions, St John's wort grows throughout Europe, flowering from the second half of June through to September. Traditionally, it was thought to flower on 24 June— St John's Eve, but is probably at its best at the end of June and in early July. It grows mainly in clumps but can be found as a single plant. An herbaceous perennial, it usually dies back to its roots each year, sending up new growth in the spring.

In its preferred habitat the plant will grow up to a maximum of about one metre (three feet) in height, each stem, which may be two-ridged, sending out alternate pairs of leaf stems. Each leaf stem from the middle upwards produces clusters of yellow-gold flowers, finely speckled, on close examination, with tiny red-black dots along the margins of the petals. The leaves close to the top of the plant also have this speckling, and the many red-black dots (hypericin oil glands, containing large amounts of this constituent) along the margins of the petals and upper leaves are one of the key distinguishing features of St John's wort (*Hypericum perforatum*). Closely related species also have these glands but in much smaller numbers; and as a rule of thumb, the greater the number of red-black glands on the plant the better it will be as a medicine.

If you hold a leaf of St John's wort up to the sun you can see why the plant was given its botanical name *'perforatum'*: the opaque, slightly white dots (oil glands) distributed across the whole of each leaf allow light through, giving the leaf a 'perforated' or slightly speckled look (see illustration).

Despite these two very specific signs, unless you know a little botany identifying St John's wort can be difficult, not least because many *Hypericum* species hybridise or cross-breed. There are at least four varieties of St John's wort (*Hypericum perforatum*) found in Europe: broad-, narrow-, intermediate- and small-leaved. The southern European narrow-leaved variety, *angustifolium*, has the greatest concentration of both types of oil glands, and is preferred as a medicine. As a rule, looking first for the red-black oil glands, and second for the 'perforated' translucent oil glands, will prove a reliable guide to identifying it as *Hypericum perforatum* or a very close relative.

However, it is easy to make mistakes when identifying plants—and some are poisonous. If you are unfamiliar with botany, you might confuse St John's wort with ragwort (*Senecio jacobea*), itself a common meadow and wayside plant. Ragwort is highly toxic to the liver and will kill cattle that graze upon it. If you have found a plant that you think is St John's wort, and you intend to use it, whether topically or internally, as an infusion or an oil, you must take proper steps to identify it accurately. If in doubt, show it to someone who is familiar with plant identification or do not use it.

Though a native of Europe, western Asia and Russia, growing almost up to the Arctic circle, St John's wort has followed European migration to Australia and New Zealand, the USA and

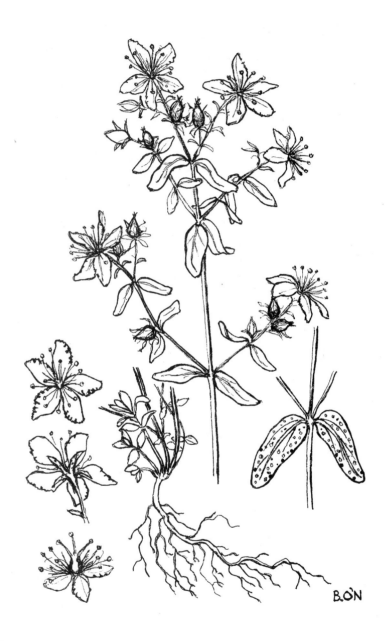

Canada. On the west coast of North America it has long been regarded as a noxious weed;[3] so much so that it was considered 'a serious problem for livestock in California during the first half of the 20th century. Sheep that foraged on St John's Wort became severely affected, with the skin on the face swelling to such an extent that the condition was referred to as "bighead". If the lips become affected, the animal is unable to feed and starves to death . . . a biological control program using beetles that feed exclusively on St John's Wort has successfully curtailed its spread.'[5]

This is an extreme description of hypericism, the photosensitisation that can occur if St John's wort is taken in very large quantities (far beyond normal medicinal dosages), and indicates that the plant is definitely not suitable as a food! Ironically, the deliberate introduction to California in 1946 of the flea beetle (*Chrysolina quadrigemina*), a heavy feeder on St John's wort, as a part of this biological programme, now complicates the possible cultivation of St John's wort as a cash crop in parts of the USA.

St John's wort in cultivation

Most commercially grown St John's wort comes from eastern Europe, though much is still wild-crafted—gathered from the wild—especially in eastern and north-western North America, and Australia. For commercial cultivation, field investigations in Poland suggest that the best time for planting the seeds is in the autumn, in rows about 30–40cm (12–15in) apart.[6]

Despite the fact that the plant can grow prolifically, a key concern with the increasing popularity of St John's wort is that wild-crafting may threaten its survival in some regions. Current commercial prices for St John's wort are around £5.50 ($9.00) per kg and rising. As with other medicinal plants, the more valuable it becomes as a commodity the more pressure there will be on it in the wild.

In the long term a responsible attitude by the consumer—that is, all those benefiting from its medicinal activity—insisting on produce that has been either cultivated or wild-crafted in an environmentally sensitive manner, is the only way to ensure that

St John's wort, and other similarly threatened wild plants, remain common in the wild. This attitude also encourages the greater availability of organically grown plant material. St John's wort, like other medicinal plants, will absorb industrial pollutants[7] and artificial pesticides, and organically certified material is always to be preferred.

In the garden, Rose of Sharon (*H. calycinum*) and Tutsan (*H. androsaemum*) are near relatives of St John's wort. Both may be used medicinally and have anti-depressant activity,[8] although Rose of Sharon does not contain hypericin. There is growing evidence that Rose of Sharon could be used in a similar way to *H. perforatum*: animal studies in Turkey suggest that an extract of Rose of Sharon may be as effective as St John's wort and the conventional anti-depressant imipramine in relieving depression. Rose of Sharon also showed some analgesic activity.[8] Both plants are larger and more bushy than St John's wort, the yellow flowers of Rose of Sharon being up to 5cm (2in) across and structurally similar to those of St John's wort. St John's wort itself can be grown as a garden plant for ornamental or medicinal reasons, as it will flourish in moderately dry soils and a sunny aspect. Its brilliant yellow flowers will add colour and light to any garden. Easy to cultivate, it is best sown in pots or a fine soil in spring or autumn. From their second year on the plants will continue to re-grow year on year and will re-seed many times over if given the chance.

Harvesting, drying and storing

Botanists have found that some plants time their growth and flowering with soil and air temperature, others by day length and the position of the sun. There can be little doubt that St John's wort falls into this latter category, for year after year it flowers towards the end of June. This has been observed since ancient times and the herb has often had magical significance in solstice festivities. Historically, the herb has always been gathered as it comes into flower; Paracelsus, the famous sixteenth-century German doctor, herbalist and chemist, maintained that St John's wort flowers should be picked at sunrise, and many herbalists continue to support this tradition. However, from a pharmacological point of view, recent investigations suggest that levels of active constituents within the plant vary throughout its flowering cycle, opening up the possibility that times of harvesting can be refined to maximise the content of different active constituents:

Flavonoids, proanthocyanidins	— highest content at budding
Hypericin, pseudohypericin, tannins	— highest content at blossoming
Hyperforin, adhyperforin	— highest content in seed capsules[2]

As the anti-depressant activity appears to be more strongly linked to the herb's hyperforin content than any other single constituent, picking the herb later in the summer when there are more seed capsules might increase its strength of activity. Whereas if one is looking for a strong antiviral action (largely due to hypericin/pseudohypericin content), then one should pick the herb as the flowers open. In practice, one can pick early on in flowering and then have a second 'crop' later in the summer, as the plant continues to flower and go to seed. It would then be interesting to compare the relative therapeutic value of each crop.

Always choose a dry, sunny morning to collect the herb. Avoid damaged, infested or diseased plants. Ensure that you are collecting St John's wort and not some other herb. Pick the flowering tops about 10–15cm (4–6in) from the top and place in an open tray or brown paper bag. For St John's wort oil the flowers, being the most therapeutically active part of the plant, are sometimes picked on their own. It is far better to grow the plant than to pick it from the wild as there is no guarantee that wild-crafted herbs are free from crop-spraying, pollution or other forms of contamination. If gathering from the wild be aware of these problems and collect only where the plant grows abundantly. Respect the plant, do *not* overpick and threaten its survival in the area. Collect only what is needed and will be used.

The herb can be used fresh as an infusion (tea) or to make St John's wort oil. If using fresh, process as soon as possible. If drying, an airing cupboard or a dry, airy but shaded room is fine. Place the herb on plain paper or hang from a line, drying it as quickly as possible. As soon as the flowering tops are dry—brittle but not bone-dry—carefully rub the flowers and leaves off the stems and place in a brown paper bag or dark glass jar. This traditional method of drying is completely acceptable but can probably be improved on, best results being obtained by drying the herb in an oven at 70°C (158°F) for 10 hours.[9] No matter how you dry the herb, make sure you store it in a cool, dry and dark place. When dried and stored properly the herb will remain medicinally useful for up to 12 months.

Natural variability

Along with most things natural, St John's wort is subject to significant variation in its growth and the constituents that it forms. Some batches of the herb will contain high levels of active constituents, for example hypericin and pseudohypericin, others quite low levels. These variations are largely unpredictable and depend not only on the variety of the herb—for example, the northern European broad-leaved variety of St John's wort, var. *perforatum*, has significantly lower hypericin levels than the southern Europe narrow-leaved var. *angustifolium*[10]—but also on ecological factors:[11] the soil, seasonal variations in rainfall and sunlight, height above sea level (flavonoid content is affected by altitude but hypericin is not), companion plants and so on. In short, in a world where quality control is ever more important, St John's wort—in common with all other herbal medicines—seems to be infuriatingly unpredictable.

Provided one has well dried, good quality plant material as a starting point, there are basically two difference approaches to this issue of variability. You can treat St John's wort as close to a foodstuff, recognising that life itself is subject to infinite variety, and in common with previous generations take the herb as nature has created it—as an organically grown product. Such an approach

31

is fine for relatively minor health problems, or where different herbs are being taken together as an infusion, but for consistent long-term use in the treatment of more serious illness, standardised preparations are probably a better bet.

By taking a pharmaceutically-tested 'standardised extract' you are theoretically guaranteed that a specific level of an identified constituent—most hypericum extracts are standardised at 0.3 per cent hypericin—is present. However, there is no guarantee that the selected constituent is the most important 'marker', and in any case the herb as a whole has greater anti-depressant activity than any one of its active constituents. Hypericin is probably the best 'marker' for the herb's *antiviral* activity, but is definitely *not* the most appropriate one for its *anti-depressant* activity—the major medicinal use of the plant. Standardised products therefore provide evidence of the quality of plant material rather than of its effectiveness, and in some cases good quality dried St John's wort may prove superior to standardised extracts, especially where specific genetic strains of the plant are grown.[12]

*　　*　　*

Recommendations on medicinal use, dosage, available preparations and buying hypericum will be found in chapter 8.

CHAPTER 3

Hypericum—Herbal Anti-depressant

Nothing chases away disease like strength. Therefore, we should seek medicines with power and strength to overcome whatever illnesses they are used against. From this it follows that God has given to Perforatum (St John's wort) the strength to chase (away) the ghosts of nature . . . and all downheartedness.

Paracelsus (1493–1541)

When in 1996 the *British Medical Journal* published an article which concluded that 'Hypericum extracts are more effective than placebo for treating mild to moderately severe depressive disorders',[1] a milestone had been reached. At last, after well over a decade of in-depth scientific research (mostly in Germany), the Anglo-American medical world was waking up to the potential benefits of hypericum in the treatment of depression. Here, if the research was right, was a herb as effective as conventional anti-depressants, which could be cultivated and produced at relatively low cost, and had a very low incidence of side-effects.

Since then, news of the medicinal value of the plant has spread around the world with demand for hypericum products soaring. Research has continued and expanded and there is now a burgeoning body of evidence to support the use of hypericum in the treatment of depressive illness. A 1998 paper, detailing a clinical trial, finished like several before it: 'Hypericum extract was shown to be an effective option in the treatment of mildly or moderately depressed patients, which avoids the well-known side-effects of other anti-depressant agents'.[2]

33

HYPERICUM

Although hypericum has many potential uses as a medicine, it is its role as an anti-depressant that has struck home, and it is not hard to see why: depression is a common and desperately difficult problem to treat, let alone to live with.

DEPRESSION

Almost everyone has experienced symptoms of depression brought on in response to life's crises, to long-term stress, to anxiety or nervous exhaustion. On this level it is part of the human condition, bringing with it at various times a loss of joy in life, a feeling of emptiness, a lack of energy, of confidence, of hope and self-esteem, difficulty in concentrating and making decisions, a sense of guilt, and if that was not enough, a whole range of symptoms affecting appetite, weight and sleep combined with aches and pains and loss of libido.

Fortunately most people do not suffer from all these symptoms at once, and in any case usually manage to throw off such feelings after a relatively short time. Such short-lived symptoms are the norm, but depression occurs across the spectrum from mild to moderate to severe. The same range of symptoms occurs in each case but at different levels of intensity. About 10 per cent of people with depressive illness suffer what is assessed as severe depression, which is often profoundly disabling, bringing with it permanently dark clouds of apathy and despair, and thoughts of suicide. Over half those who attempt suicide are suffering from depressive illness.

Awareness of the damaging effects of depression is not new, and authors from ancient Greece onwards have described depressive symptoms and behaviour with great acuity. One Greek physician, Soranus of Ephesus (c. AD 100), detailed the signs of 'melancholy' as:

> mental anguish and distress, dejection, silence, animosity toward members of the household, sometimes a desire to live and at other times a longing for death, suspicion on the part

of the patient that a plot is being hatched against him, weeping without reason, and occasional joviality.[3]

Whilst emotional and practical support, care and love—'unconditional love is life's most powerful medicine'[4]—are always likely to be the most important factors in aiding recovery from depressive illness, medicines that prove effective in treating or alleviating depression are big news, especially when one considers the vast numbers of people affected. Between 3 and 5 per cent of the world's population are thought to suffer from depressive illness,[5] with well over a hundred million people probably affected at any one time and women suffering about twice as often as men. In the developed West the incidence appears to be higher, with over 17 million adults in the USA affected, costing $44 billion in treatment, disability and lost productivity.[5] In the UK it affects 2.8 million people at any one time. In Australia, 10 per cent of the population are thought to suffer symptoms of sufficient severity and duration to be diagnosed as suffering a depressive illness,[6] while figures in other Western countries are at a similar or higher level and showing alarming signs of increase.[7] The scale of depressive illness indicated by these figures, and the misery entailed, are almost unimaginable. Little wonder that treatments which appear to offer benefit are seized on by both the medical profession and the public and, like Prozac, become household names.

Hypericum as an anti-depressant

Hypericum is a safe and effective anti-depressant, usually taking about two to three weeks of treatment[8] before improvement is noted. People report a subtle but steady lightening of mood, and a lifting of many of the other symptoms of depression. Sleep improves and some people experience increased energy levels. It appears to improve motivation, concentration and emotional stability. In some clinical trials, it improved memory and 'cognitive function'.

Hypericum has by now been so well researched that one can ask why it is not yet a standard treatment for depression in English-speaking countries in the way that it is in Germany. Different people, it seems, demand different levels of proof! That said, scepticism about claims for new 'wonder' treatments for depression is justified, for depression is a condition which frequently responds to treatment in any form. In clinical trials of anti-depressants, somewhere between 10 and 40 per cent of patients, given not the drug but placebos, improve! To show that a medicine really does work as an anti-depressant and that the positive effect is over and above that of the placebo, you therefore need to show that it works for 60–80 per cent of patients taking it.[9] By way of making the point more strongly, a recent article in the *New Scientist* suggested that much of the activity of Prozac may be due to the side-effects it produces, suggesting that some of the hype surrounding the drug may be just that.[10] Put baldly, people taking Prozac appear to gain confidence that the treatment is working precisely because the drug's side-effects *make them feel worse*! If they feel worse, then the drug must be effective, and thus they feel greater certainty that they are improving. Hypericum, with its low level of side-effects, obviously does not stand a chance when competing in this kind of ball game.

It is true that hypericum is not yet as intensively researched as a newly developed synthetic anti-depressant would need to be, nor is there clear evidence yet that it is appropriate for severe depressive illness. But hypericum is not a laboratory-based drug being put on the market for the first time. It is a medicinal plant with a history of traditional use for nervous problems, including depression, dating back over two thousand years, and with a very low incidence of side-effects at a therapeutic dosage (for details of contra-indications, interactions and side-effects, see chapter 8).

On top of the 23 double-blind or open clinical trials involving 1,757 patients reviewed by Linde *at al.* in the *BMJ* article (1996),[1] a further three major trials have since been published, each finding positive results for hypericum. At least 16 trials have also been conducted on healthy volunteers. The European monograph on hypericum, produced by the European Scientific Cooperative for Phytotherapy,[11] states that clinical trials have shown 'a significant improvement of (the) main symptoms (of depression)—mood, loss of interest and activity, and other symptoms—sleep, concentration, somatic complaints'.

A 'drug-monitoring study' involving 3,250 patients produced fairly typical results: 82 per cent of doctors and 79 per cent of patients assessed the outcome as between 'better' and 'symptom free', with around 15 per cent noting no change or 'worse'. Forty-seven patients (1.45 per cent) withdrew from treatment due to digestive problems or allergic reactions[12] (see chapter 8 for side-effects recorded).

Most trials have compared the effects of hypericum extract (mostly Jarsin/LI160, produced by Lichtwer Pharma) with placebo, with hypericum on average being about twice as effective as placebo.[1] Where hypericum extracts have been compared to conventional anti-depressants the results again on average indicate that the extract is slightly more effective than the drug being compared, e.g. imipramine, maprotiline. Almost all these comparative trials conclude that hypericum is as effective as conventional anti-depressants, and that due to its low incidence of side-effects it is a preferred treatment in mild to moderate depression. One recent six-week trial undertaken at the Royal Masonic Hospital in London[13] concluded that 'since side-effects are the most important limiting factor for patient compliance, Hypericum extracts offer the possibility to treat patients more adequately with anti-depressant pharmacotherapy'.

These 'averaged-out' results referred to above do hide a number of problems with the clinical trials, which include: a wide variation in assessing the severity of depression in the patients on the trial; a lack of long-term studies—most trials have lasted only four or six weeks; and the low dosage of conventional anti-depressants used in comparison with hypericum. These and other weaknesses have been identified by Linde *et al.*[1] Clinical trials undertaken since 1996 have by and large taken these criticisms into account— and the results continue to confirm the value of hypericum extracts in relieving depression.

Whether or not hypericum is effective for severe depression is a still unanswered question. However, used at double the standard dosage (1,800mg a day of standardised extract), hypericum extract proved more or less as effective as imipramine in treating severe depression, with over 60 per cent of patients rating hypericum as 'very good' or 'good'. Side-effects were considerably lower than in the imipramine group, despite the high daily dosage of hypericum. The clinicians noted that hypericum should not be restricted to mild to moderate depression only, as severely depressed patients could also benefit from it.[14]

Perhaps the best proof of hypericum's efficacy, however, lies elsewhere—in the literally millions of people who are self-medicating for depression, either trying hypericum as the first line of treatment or actively switching from a synthetic anti-depressant to hypericum. Why? Obviously, because it seems to be effective for mild to moderate depression and causes significantly fewer side-effects. But perhaps also because, as medical herbalists have always thought, hypericum is not just an anti-depressant, a medication that relieves depression: it also acts to restore and strengthen the nervous system as a whole. Depression is often due to nervous exhaustion, adrenal 'burn-out' or viral infection. Hypericum's activity in relieving anxiety and insomnia, and in countering certain viral infections, directly complements its anti-depressant activity, encouraging a return to health. Given that the herb also enhances performance in athletes, one cannot help wondering whether it is not a tonic for both body and mind.

What causes depression?

As one might expect, current scientific theories of depression mostly focus on the bodily (biochemical) aspects of the condition. These theories throw significant light on how hypericum acts as an anti-depressant at a cellular level and within the brain, but they do not generally provide a rounded or holistic view of depression or of the activity of hypericum extracts in treating it. The development over the last ten years of a theory that links depression with the immune system, however, offers the strong possibility of integrating the biochemical and the psychological factors involved in depression. The following sections give a brief summary of the different theories put forward to explain the mechanisms involved in depression.

The monoamine theory

The billions of neurones within the brain communicate with each other mainly by chemical messengers known as neurotransmitters. These are released from one neurone into the synapse (or space) between it and an adjoining neurone. When the neurotransmitter 'locks on' to a receptor on the surface of this second neurone the message is delivered and the nerve impulse is communicated across the synapse from one cell to the next. Some of these neurotransmitters—serotonin, noradrenaline (norepinephrine) and dopamine, all of them *monoamines*—are important in maintaining a positive mood, and lowered levels, which lead to reduced nervous activity, are linked to depressive illness. This is the basis of the monoamine theory of depression, perhaps the key biochemical explanation of the disorder, whereby depression is thought to be caused principally by deficient levels of serotonin and noradrenaline.

There are, however, a number of problems with this theory. Firstly, it is really no more than an explanation of the observed action of drugs commonly used to treat depression. Imipramine, a 'tricyclic' anti-depressant, for example, maintains monoamine levels within the synapse by reducing the rate of breakdown of the neurotransmitter; Prozac (fluoxetine) on the other hand is a 'selective serotonin reuptake inhibitor' (SSRI), which maintains serotonin levels within the synapse by preventing their removal into the cell. Secondly, although anti-depressant drugs do increase neurotransmitter levels—by inhibiting their removal from the synapse (or their breakdown once reabsorbed)—this effect occurs rapidly, while the anti-depressant effect for which they are being taken takes several weeks to develop, typically about 3–4 weeks. The conclusion therefore is that other factors, besides changes in monoamine levels, are involved in the onset of depression. These other factors are slowly and very sketchily being linked together. In particular, a deeper understanding of how the nervous and the immune systems work together—the field of psychoneuroimmun-ology—is opening up the way for a far more comprehensive theory of depression.

The immune system theory

It is now known beyond doubt that the brain and the immune system communicate with each other in a complex two-way process that includes chemical messengers such as cytokines (immune system 'transmitters'), steroid hormones and neurotransmitters.[15] Cytokines are released by large circulating white blood cells (known as macrophages) whenever an immune response is triggered—usually by the presence of a threat to normal cellular life, such as viral infection. Once released, many cytokines stimulate inflammation *within* the body, causing heat, swelling and tenderness. At the same time cytokines act *within* the brain to stimulate the release of a whole series of neurotransmitters and steroid hormones, especially cortisol, which together damp down and control the strength of the inflammatory 'response', for if inflammation is left uncontrolled within the body it has devastating effects. It is this damping, negative feedback mechanism that is thought to be a significant factor in the onset of depression. The cytokines most involved in this process are interleukin-1 and -6 (IL-1 and IL-6) and tumour necrosis factor-alpha (TNF-α). IL-1 and IL-6, in particular, stimulate the release of corticotrophin-releasing hormone (CRH) within the hypothalamus, the area of the brain most involved in emotion, mood and auto-regulation.[16]

In turn, increased CRH levels lead eventually, via the body's main stress pathway—known as the hypothalamic-pituitary-adrenal axis (HPA)—to the increased release of steroid hormones from the adrenal gland, especially cortisol (hydrocortisone). Cortisol has a very powerful anti-inflammatory action within the body, and high levels of CRH and cortisol are common findings in patients suffering from depressive illness. Furthermore, high levels of cortisol—triggered by stress as well as by inflammation—appear to directly reduce levels of serotonin, noradrenaline and dopamine within the brain . . . which leads in turn to the onset of depression.

Connections can therefore be made that link up many of the processes involved in depression, connections that also throw light on how hypericum works as an anti-depressant. It is clear that a whole range of chemical messengers, including monoamines, cytokines, CRH, pituitary hormones and adrenal hormones, all interact in specific and complex ways to produce depression. Of equal importance, it becomes possible to connect the biochemical changes involved in depression with what is happening on an emotional and psychological level. Everyone knows on a common-sense level that a depressed mood, negative thinking and high stress levels can create the situation where depressive illness (in the biochemical sense) takes hold. The immune (or macrophage) theory of depression begins—very sketchily—to explain how this comes about (see diagram p. 42), and indicates that treatment for depression should always be considered on both an emotional and biochemical level.

Despite the elegance of this theory, it is a far from complete explanation of how depression occurs, and two further factors need to be added in before we can start to look at hypericum's role as an anti-depressant.

The 'GABA' theory
There is yet another theory of depression—this time linked mostly with anxiety and stress. Benzodiazepine drugs such as Valium have been used extensively since the 1960s to suppress and relieve anxiety and panic. In recent years they have become less popular as they are strongly addictive. Nevertheless, research is now showing that certain benzodiazepine drugs can be used successfully to treat depressive illness.[17] As a consequence, scientists are asking how such drugs produce this effect and how a drug that has a sedative action can help in depression. It has been known for a while that benzodiazepines do indirectly increase γ-amino butyric acid (GABA) levels within the brain, strengthening this neurotransmitter's 'tranquillising' activity. The suggestion is now that in certain areas of the brain (the prefrontal cortex and hippocampus) stimulation of GABA levels, which is what benzodiazepines do,

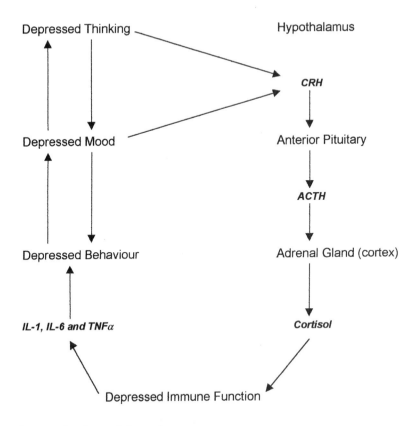

Immune function and depression.
Depressed mood and thinking can alter neuroendocrine, and subsequently immune, function. Likewise, depressed immune function and behaviour can induce depressed moods, thought and brain function.
(Adapted from Watkins, A. (ed.), *Mind-Body Medicine*, Churchill Livingstone, 1997. Reproduced by permission.)

leads to an increase in noradrenaline levels. In other words, benzodiazepines indirectly stimulate monoamine levels, suggesting a further pathway by which monoamine levels may be raised and an anti-depressant effect produced. As there is evidence that hypericum relieves anxiety as well as depression, this particular mechanism may be important in explaining how the herb works as an anti-depressant.

Melatonin and depression

Finally, and you could be forgiven at this point for wondering whether this is a book on hypericum or on brain chemistry, one more neuro-transmitter needs to be thrown into the equation—melatonin. Melatonin is a poorly-understood hormone produced by the pineal gland, which lies at the base of the brain. It is involved in maintaining regular body rhythms and is released more when there is less daylight—during the winter months in the northern and southern hemispheres. It has been observed that melatonin levels are often abnormal in people suffering from depression, and are deficient in seasonal effective disorder (SAD). It now seems likely that raised CRH levels within the brain inhibit the release of melatonin from the pineal gland,[18] a finding that gives further weight to the depressive role of CRH within the central nervous system and the body as a whole. Melatonin and serotonin also appear to inhibit each other.

*   *   *

The reason for having gone into such detail in looking at the bio-chemical processes linked to depression is that they help to explain how hypericum works in depression, as well as in anxiety, seasonal affective disorder, nervous exhaustion and other related problems.

HOW DOES HYPERICUM WORK?

The development of the scientific understanding of how hypericum works as an anti-depressant is a little like reading a good detective story. As each gripping chapter comes to an end, a different and previously unsuspected character appears as the figure most likely to be responsible for the crime that has been committed. The key difference of course is that in hypericum's case this particular detective story is still very much in progress and no one is yet able to point the finger with absolute confidence at any one of a number of suspects. In fact, on the basis of current evidence, a number of suspects will end up being held jointly responsible for the herb's anti-depressant activity—more a group conspiracy than an individual act!

The previous 'form' or record of the active constituents within St John's wort led researchers initially to focus their efforts on three key groups of constituents: the napthodianthrones—hypericin and pseudohypericin; the flavonoids—a large and varied group of constituents including xanthones; and the phloroglucinols—hyperforin and adhyperforin. Other constituents in the running included the essential oil.

A brief history—from MAOI to GABA!

Investigations into St John's wort started a long time ago—in fact hypericin was first isolated from the herb in 1830 by the German chemist Buchner.[19] Only since the late 1970s, however, has research focused on identifying the active constituent(s) responsible for the herb's activity as an anti-depressant and the way in which this effect is achieved.

Initially, hypericin was the key suspect, being thought to work by inhibiting MAO.[20] However, this result was shown to be an error due to using 80 per cent pure hypericin in the investigations, for it emerged that pure hypericin has almost no MAOI activity at all ('Using pure hypericin no relevant inhibiting factors could be shown'[21]). The answer must therefore lie in the remaining 20 per cent. Suspicion fell on the xanthones which have MAOI-type activity in isolation,[22, 23] but it was shown that such small amounts occur within the plant that this group could not in itself be responsible. At the same time the finger was pointed at the flavonoids, clearly one of the most important groups of constituents within the plant.[21] These do appear to have an MAOI activity but at a relatively low level, and in any case they have no 'form'—despite being widespread in the plant world there was little record of them having significant anti-depressant activity in other plants. In any case, at about the same time the whole idea that St John's wort worked principally by inhibiting MAO began to be thrown into doubt.[24, 25] Eventually it emerged that St John's wort does have an MAOI-type activity, as well as an effect on catechol-omethyltransferase (COMT)—another enzyme that breaks down monoamine neurotransmitters—but at such a weak level that 'the clinically proven anti-depressive effect of hypericum extracts cannot be explained in terms of MAO inhibition'.[21]

So if hypericum does not work by inhibiting the breakdown of monoamine neurotransmitters such as serotonin, how does it work? A 1995 paper concluded that 'Hypericum extract displays its anti-depressant activity via an inhibition of serotonin uptake by postsynaptic receptors.'[25] In other words, hypericum extracts work in a manner not too dissimilar to Prozac and other SSRIs. This was now the favoured explanation, though the constituents responsible had yet to be identified, and serious doubts were raised by researchers that sufficiently high concentrations were achieved at normal therapeutic dosages for an SSRI-type effect to be responsible for the herb's anti-depressant action.

Other 'leads' put forward at this time and still to be followed up include the suggestion that a GABA-type activity might be involved.[26] Swiss research has indicated that amentoflavone, a flavonoid, may have a benzodiazepine-type effect.[27]

As research has expanded it has become clear that hypericum extracts affect not only serotonin levels but noradrenaline and dopamine as well.[24] Furthermore, it appears that 'the fact that hypericum shows a similar affinity for three different neurotransmitter transporter systems might point to an unique and not yet known mechanism of inhibition of neurotransmitter uptake.' In other words, because hypericum has such a wide-ranging effect on these monoamines it may exert its anti-depressant effect by an as yet unknown process.[24] Indeed, research into the herb's mode of action, like research into other medicinal plants—for example, *Ginkgo biloba*—is likely to lead to a new and deeper understanding of the functioning of neurotransmitters and the central nervous system in general.

Hyperforin—the overlooked player?
The story now continues with an unexpected twist. A previously overlooked constituent—hyperforin—has been put forward as the

most likely candidate for hypericum's anti-depressant activity, and the evidence is fairly compelling. It had long been assumed that hyperforin, which has a powerful anti-microbial activity, was too unstable to be a key player in this area. Furthermore, most German research has been funded by companies producing hypericin-standardised extracts. One consequence of this is that the vast majority of clinical trials have used hypericin-standardised extracts, and only recently have experiments been conducted on alternative hypericum preparations. Research published in 1998 has finally shown that a hyperforin-rich extract (using a CO_2 extraction process) is significantly more anti-depressant than hypericin-standardised extracts.[24]

Hyperforin has been shown to be readily bioavailable, to be able to cross the blood brain barrier (i.e. to get in to the brain), and to have a distinct anti-depressant activity in its own right— probably a serotonin uptake inhibition,[28] though it equally affects noradrenaline, dopamine and GABA levels.[29] Hyperforin does indeed seem to be the leading actor in producing an anti-depressant effect, *though it requires a supporting act.* 'Our results indicate that hyperforin is a major, but not the only, anti-depressant or centrally active component'; and later, '*Hypericum perforatum* is a further example of a traditional herbal drug which does not contain a single active principle or one specific mechanism of action.'[24]

As a herbal practitioner I breathe a sigh of relief on reading these words. Here is a sign that the complexity of natural medicines is beginning to be acknowledged (and scientifically confirmed). Just as important, there is growing recognition that many medicinal plants—for example, garlic (*Allium sativum*)—work by the *combined action* of a number of relatively weak effects on the body. In St John's wort's case, none of the active constituents alone produces as strong an anti-depressant action as extracts of the whole plant, and the clinical efficacy of hypericum is clearly the consequence of the combined contribution of several mechanisms—each one too weak by itself to account for the overall effect.

Summary

The biochemical effects that hypericum produces on the central nervous system are remarkably wide-ranging. It markedly increases, to a significant degree, serotonin, noradrenaline and dopamine levels within the synapse, and seems to enhance the tranquillising activity of GABA and benzodiazepine—all of which are involved, as discussed above, in the onset or maintenance of depression. The ways in which hypericum acts on levels of these neurotransmitters is complex, but as a rule the effects correspond with the results one would expect to see from treatment with conventional drugs such as 'tricyclic' anti-depressants, and from SSRIs such as Prozac.

At the same time, hypericum extracts have been shown to have a potent effect on cytokine levels, especially IL-1, IL-6 and TNF-α, which stimulate CRH release within the hypothalamus, leading to significantly raised cortisol levels in the body. B. Thiele and co-workers (1994)[30] explored the ability of a hypericum extract (LI160) to suppress IL-6 release from a whole human blood culture. The extract was found to cause 'a massive suppression of interleukin-6 release'. This study was *in vitro* (in isolated tissue in a test-tube), but were such effects to be repeated *in vivo* (in living subjects), this would go a long way to support the theory that hypericum achieves its anti-depressant effect at least in part by an immune suppressant or anti-inflammatory activity.

It is also possible that the plant has a direct effect on melatonin levels, which are often lowered in depressive illness. The herb actually contains small amounts of melatonin,[31] though it is doubtful that this manages to bypass the liver in significant quantities. It appears that while CRH inhibits melatonin release, melatonin for its part (like GABA) inhibits CRH release. Here, perhaps, is another route through which hypericum can influence depressive states.

Finally, since beginning to write this chapter, there are signs that hypericum might influence levels of pain-killing opiates in the central nervous system. In laboratory experiments, hypericum extracts had a strong affinity for opioid receptors that trigger pain relief, and this could be yet another route by which the herb achieves its anti-depressant activity.[32]

To summarise, research to date indicates that hypericum may work by influencing levels of the following neurotransmitters and hormones:

- Serotonin, noradrenaline and dopamine
- MAO, COMT
- GABA
- Melatonin
- CRH, cortisol

New and unexpected findings will certainly be made in coming years, as the research already underway continues to expand. However, given the extreme complexity of the processes underlying depression, and the ways in which hypericum acts upon them, it is unlikely that a single explanation will emerge for a very long time, if at all. What will become clearer is the type of depression, and perhaps the type of individual, that responds best to treatment with hypericum. Extracts of the herb can then be used in a more precise manner. In the meantime, people can take hypericum for mild to moderate depression, and for many of the unpleasant symptoms accompanying it, in the knowledge that it is a safe and effective remedy.

OTHER RELATED USES OF ST JOHN'S WORT

Attempts to understand how the central nervous system works, and how it interacts with hormonal and immune function, are as complicated an area of study as one could imagine. It is very largely unmapped territory, although some brave souls have recently attempted to sketch its outlines. These are probably as accurate as mediaeval maps of the world—that is highly inaccurate—but they are nonetheless the best guides that exist and do help in trying to bring together hypericum's different medicinal actions.

Although so little is known about the workings of the central nervous system, following the current understanding of the role of serotonin, it seems very likely that hypericum has a range of therapeutically valuable uses directly linked to its ability to influence serotonin levels, as well as those of other neurotransmitters.

Serotonin in particular is regarded as the key neurotransmitter in a vast range of emotional and psychiatric problems, and 'has taken the centre stage in the last few years: it appears to regulate sleep and appetite.'[33] Some authors go much farther, and argue that disordered serotonin metabolism is linked with an astonishing array of mental and other health problems, including 'addictions, attention deficit disorder, chronic pain, depression, dysthmia, eating disorders, headache, obsessive-compulsive disorders, panic, poor impulse control, post-traumatic stress disorders, premenstrual syndrome, sleep disorders, stress disorders, sudden cardiac death and violence'.[34]

This list may be a good example of overstating one's case, but setting aside sudden cardiac death and violence, it has an uncanny resemblance to many of St John's wort's uses in herbal medicine. With this list in mind it is possible to move out from the core area of understanding of the herb—as an anti-depressant—and to look at potential uses which, though not as scientifically established, nonetheless tend to conform with the herb's long-standing traditional use in Western herbal medicine.

Seasonal affective disorder

Seasonal affective disorder (SAD) has a lot in common with depression, so it is not surprising that St John's wort can be helpful in easing this condition. Almost everyone knows the 'winter blues' and instinctively feels more cheerful in bright, sunny weather. The amount of light, especially sunlight, that we are exposed to has a direct link with how we feel. During the winter months, with their long nights and short days, reduced light levels can lead to a sense of gloom and despondency, and it is not fanciful to imagine St John's wort, flowering as it does around midsummer, as a kind of stored natural 'sunlight' for the 'winter blues'. Indeed, as a herb that both affects sensitivity to light and lightens mood, it would be surprising if it failed to ease gloomy, sunless conditions such as SAD.

SAD itself is really a more extreme version of the 'winter blues', typically beginning in October or November, with symptoms that include lack of energy, depressed mood, anxiety, loss of concentration and of libido, sleeping long hours and weight gain. It is clearly linked to light levels, for the farther from the equator you travel the higher the incidence of SAD—particularly in the far north where major seasonal mood variation has been shown to occur throughout the whole population.[35] In the UK, an estimated one million people a year are affected.

In normal circumstances, reduced exposure to light leads to increased release from the pineal gland of melatonin, the hormone which circulates in the body, adjusting life to the basic rhythm of night and day.[36] In those with SAD lower levels are released and this is thought to be the biochemical basis of the disorder. Lowered melatonin levels are often associated with depressive illness, and SAD can on one level be seen as seasonal depression. First-line treatment for SAD is often with artificial sunlight rather than drug therapy, and patients usually respond well to light treatment (phototherapy).

As mentioned above, there are signs that melatonin levels are reduced by CRH,[35] and that serotonin levels play a key role in melatonin regulation. Hypericum contains relatively high concentrations of melatonin,[31] and as the pineal gland lies outside the blood-brain barrier which normally stops all but small molecules from entering the brain, melatonin could be a further active constituent within hypericum contributing to its overall therapeutic value.

In healthy volunteers, an intravenous hypericum extract reduced the amount of light needed to suppress melatonin release, and night-time levels of melatonin increased significantly after medication.[22] Another study of 20 patients concluded that hypericum was useful in treating the depressive aspects of SAD and, unexpectedly, that light therapy did not add greatly to its effectiveness.[35]

Although not yet fully substantiated, the indications are that

St John's wort is an effective treatment for SAD, well worth trying as self-treatment in non-severe cases. The closeness of SAD to depression, the safety and low level of side-effects of hypericum, and the logic of self-medication for such a condition—starting perhaps in the middle to end of September (i.e. when fully well)—all mean that the herb can be recommended as a first-line treatment for SAD. If it is unsuccessful after, say, four to six weeks, other treatment can be started. Light treatment can be used at the same time as St John's wort—at normal doses of hypericum extract there is no evidence of damage to the retina during light therapy. Alternatively, one can consult a herbal practitioner or naturopath who will be likely to prescribe St John's wort along with other herbs, specifically tailored to the individual's needs.

Anxiety, panic and nervous exhaustion
Although hypericum's use in anxiety is not as well substantiated as its use in depression, one can nonetheless be pretty confident that it will ease anxiety. In Western herbal medicine hypericum has always been thought of as a sedative and prescribed for certain types of anxiety, panic and stress. While other herbs are usually chosen in preference for straightforward anxiety—for example, valerian (*Valeriana officinalis*), lemon balm (*Melissa officinalis*), scullcap (*Scutellaria laterifolia*)—hypericum is often the herb of choice for anxiety states associated with nervous exhaustion. Scientific evidence backing up this mainly empirical experience also suggests that hypericum is a medicine worth considering for chronic anxiety, panic and nervous exhaustion.

In fact, given the major overlap that exists between the symptoms of anxiety and depression, and the fact that chronic stress and anxiety can lead to depressive illness, it would be surprising if St John's wort had no ability to relieve anxiety. Three clinical trials in the 1980s examined the anti-anxiety or anxiolytic effects of hypericum extracts. The first trial compared the effects of a combination of hypericum and valerian, a European medicinal plant well known for its ability to relieve anxiety, with diazepam (Valium, a benzodiazepine), at the time a very commonly prescribed tranquilliser. A hundred outpatients with symptoms of anxiety were randomly given the herbal formulation or diazepam. After two weeks of treatment the herbal preparation showed significantly greater efficacy than diazepam.[37] Though diazepam's use as an anxiolytic has declined dramatically over the last decade due to its strongly addictive nature, this does not detract from the trial's outcome—that the hypericum and valerian extract proved the better medicine.

A second double-blind trial compared hypericum extract, this time on its own, with bromazepam (a benzodiazepine similar to diazepam). After four weeks both groups of patients showed substantial improvement, but those taking hypericum had fewer side-effects and experienced improved sleep quality, self-esteem and performance.[38] In many ways the third trial, this time against placebo, is the most interesting because it investigated the effects of hypericum on 40 highly fearful patients who were also suffering from depression. Over the four weeks of treatment fear levels reduced to normal and associated symptoms of depression improved.[39]

There is a clue here that hypericum may be an appropriate remedy when anxiety is underpinned by fear rather than worry, overactivity and excessive demands. Moreover, fear and suppressed anger are emotions that many would see as linked to the onset of depression. Psychiatrists talk about learnt submission, in which apathy and passivity take the place of fear and anger, as one aspect of depression. In relieving the sensation, the fear and its damaging effects, hypericum might be acting to prevent the onset of depression.

Other factors also indicate that hypericum has real ability to soothe anxiety and panic. Several active constituents within the herb have a benzodiazepine-type effect, slowing the nervous overactivity that is so much a hallmark of anxiety. Hyperforin has an anxiolytic action in the short term, which appears to be replaced with an anti-depressant activity in the longer term,[40] and one of its breakdown products, 2-methylbutenol, is strongly sedative. The biflavone amentoflavone has also been shown to have a similar effect to diazepam in binding to benzodiazepine receptors.[27] Interestingly, all these compounds occur only in the buds, flowers and fruits of the herb.

So hypericum clearly has value in the treatment of anxiety states, either on its own or more probably in combination with valerian. Certainly, anyone suffering from anxiety and facing the choice of taking a benzodiazepine or hypericum/valerian, would be well advised to try the herbal combination first. Hypericum may also have an even wider use, perhaps in the treatment of hyperactivity or attention deficit disorder—a common problem in children— and in obsessive-compulsive disorder, a condition in which people feel impelled to repeatedly perform certain actions, such as checking to see that the doors of a house are locked. Both of these conditions involve nervous overactivity and disordered serotonin metabolism.

Insomnia

Nothing more insidiously undermines health than lack of good quality sleep. Deprive people of sleep for more than a few days and their ability to function normally, to work efficiently, to resist infection and to remain emotionally stable rapidly declines. Anxiety and depression disrupt sleep in different ways, but in each case the sleeplessness they cause acts as a vicious circle, further weakening the individual's chances of regaining mental and emotional balance.

Short-term sleep disturbances brought on by anxiety, overwork and stressful life events in general typically cause one to be overaroused and unable to switch off, lying awake in bed with a 'spinning head', and tossing from side to side unable to make the transition into restful sleep. Such disturbances are common but normally ease after a few days or weeks. St John's wort is unlikely to be a key treatment in this type of insomnia. Valerian (*Valeriana officinalis*), passion flower (*Passiflora incarnata*) and limeflowers (*Tilia* spp.) are probably more useful herbs in such a situation, having an immediate effect: they reduce restlessness and overactivity and allow the mind to slow down and switch off. Valerian in particular has been shown to improve sleep quality and does not usually cause drowsiness on waking in the morning.

That being said, there are a number of pieces of research which indicate that hypericum may have some use in the treatment of insomnia linked to anxiety, panic and fear. One comparative trial, mentioned in the previous section, used a combined mixture of valerian and hypericum, finding the combination significantly more effective than diazepam (Valium) in relieving the symptoms of anxiety (which often includes sleep disturbance),[37] while in several other trials hypericum extract on its own improved sleep quality[39, 41] by lengthening the time spent in deep sleep (divided into stages III and IV), even though in some cases actual sleep time[42] was reduced. Alongside this activity, problems associated with depression such as low self-esteem and apathy also improved.

In fact, hypericum's value in sleep disorders seems to be much more closely linked to its role in treating depression than its milder anxiolytic activity. People suffering from depression often have fitful sleep and wake in the early morning, finding it difficult if not impossible to return to sleep. There is that sinking, hopeless feeling that most people have experienced at some time, and the quality of the sleep, when it comes, is poor. One can see this as a sign of nervous underactivity in much the same way that anxiety is a sign of overactivity. It is in this depressed kind of sleep that St John's wort is likely to be most helpful, though it may well take two or more weeks to have significant effect.

Indeed, one can draw the conclusion that hypericum is not a sedative as such but exerts a tranquillising effect. In a double blind, placebo-controlled study of sleep patterns in a group of older volunteers (average 59.8 years), hypericum extract had no sedative effect, produced an increase in slow-wave brain activity which indicates time spent in deep sleep, and did not increase sleeping time—curiously, all effects *opposite* to the typical response to 'tricyclic' anti-depressants.[42] This indicates that hypericum improves sleep quality, specifically the restful deep sleep necessary to restore and maintain balanced mental and emotional activity. Significantly, increased time in Stage IV deep sleep appears to lead to increased serotonin and endorphin levels within the brain.[34] As increased serotonin levels are thought to produce better sleep,[34] one can speculate that a 'virtuous circle' might be set up here—better quality sleep reduces levels of depression, and in turn reduced depression leads to better sleep! It is also significant that the amount of time spent each night in deep, restful sleep decreases with age, while at the same time levels of depression increase. Hypericum may therefore be therapeutically useful to older people with poor quality sleep, whether or not they are suffering from identifiable depressive illness.

Unlike most treatments for insomnia, hypericum should be taken normally through the day. There is probably little to be gained by taking a higher dose in the evening before going to bed. The indications are that the standard dose is appropriate, but where insomnia rather than depression is the key problem, my guess is that a combination of St John's wort and valerian is likely to prove more effective than St John's wort on its own.

Menopausal problems
Hypericum has long been considered an effective herb for meno-pausal problems, not because it has a direct hormonal action, but because the menopause occurs at a time when women are often chronically exhausted, after several decades of working and/or bringing up a family. On top of this tiredness, the major hormonal changes that take place during menopause can present themselves as a further burden on an already overtaxed body. Nervous exhaus-tion, loss of self-confidence and arthritic aches and pains as well as menopausal symptoms such as hot flushes and poor sleep, can coincide to make life hard to bear. For women who are mothers, this is also the time when children are likely to be leaving home, creating a void in life that can be very hard to fill.

Hypericum is not a panacea for menopausal problems, nor is it an herbal alternative to HRT; nevertheless, it can bring significant relief where nervous exhaustion and depression compound the physiological changes that are taking place.

The *British Herbal Pharmacopoeia* 1983 lists menopausal

depression as the specific indication for hypericum. As Simon Mills, a leading British herbalist, writes, 'the modern practitioner still finds advantage in treating menopausal problems primarily as symptoms of depletion, requiring restorative and convalescent measures. St John's wort seems to have an ideal balance of qualities for this task.'[43] It is not difficult to see that St John's wort will lighten the load when exhaustion and depression occur at the menopause. Though this aspect of its use has not been investigated in detail, there can be little doubt that here is a herb that will have a directly beneficial effect in relieving problems connected with the menopause.

In fact, one can go one better and take St John's wort with black cohosh (*Cimicifuga racemosa*), a combination of herbs that can have a dramatic effect in relieving many of the health problems associated with the menopause. Details of the research into this valuable herbal combination are given in chapter 7.

Addictions

It's only a whisper at the moment, but there are signs that hypericum may be a help to those struggling with addiction, by supporting the process of withdrawal, stimulating cleansing within the liver and gall-bladder, and possibly protecting the liver itself. In fact, most herbalists would immediately think of hypericum when supporting a patient through 'detox', for it has always been seen as a herb that nourishes and strengthens the nervous system. St John's wort was used in a Russian study treating alcoholics suffering from both depression and peptic ulceration.[44] The 57 patients involved took regular infusions of the herb and received psychotherapy over a two-month period. Treatment was found to be effective on both counts. Others have considered its potential in treating alcoholism[45] and it is not hard to see why the herb could prove to be very helpful here—anti-depressant, and to a lesser extent, anti-anxiety activity, combined with wound-healing properties within the stomach (usually damaged in alcoholism), and improved detoxifying and perhaps protective effects on the liver, together add up to a formidable and well-targeted list.

In my own experience in aiding patients in withdrawal from tranquilliser addiction (e.g. Valium), St John's wort combined with herbs such as valerian (see chapter 7) has often proved helpful. New Zealand herbalist and pharmacist Phil Rasmussen, who has had extensive experience in aiding patients withdrawing from benzodiazepine tranquillisers, uses hypericum frequently and describes it as an anti-depressant, liver protector and nervous tonic.[46]

Though no definitive evidence exists, if taken as part of a structured regime to aid withdrawal from alcohol and drug dependence, hypericum is very likely to provide valuable support (taken at the standard dose). As with its other therapeutic uses, such treatment would need to be long term for maximum effect.

*   *   *

FOOTNOTE: Many of the studies referred to in this chapter, and elsewhere in the book, have involved animal experimentation. The best way to assess hypericum's value as a medicine, especially as an anti-depressant, is to undertake more clinical trials using human volunteers. The success of hypericum as an anti-depressant is directly due to these human studies. Some of the experiments which mice and rats have been forced to undergo in developing knowledge of depressive illness, and of hypericum's effect on it, involve cruelty. I am not against animal experimentation *per se*, but I am against a system that requires cruelty towards animals in order for a medicine with a 2,500-year history to be accepted as safe and effective. Does such experimentation do anything to create a world where depression is less likely to occur?

CHAPTER 4

Hypericum and Viral Infection

To farmers, hypericum is a pest and noxious weed. In sunny weather animals grazing on it in sufficiently large quantities can develop blistering, similar to severe sunburn. If left untended, affected animals can die from starvation due to the severe swelling of the lips that the combination of herb and sunlight produces. It has long been known that only light-coated animals are affected in this way, and if moved out of the light into a dark barn they will usually recover quite quickly.[1] These sunburn-like symptoms are a direct consequence of high levels of hypericin within the animal. Remarkably, this increased sensitivity to sunlight, or photosensitising effect, which has caused so much damage to livestock in areas as far afield as California and New South Wales, is the factor largely responsible for hypericum's potent antiviral activity. Sunlight has been shown to strongly enhance its ability to kill viruses, and scientists are now investigating the potential of combining hypericin and light to treat certain types of cancer—triggering hypericin's photosensitising effect by pulsing bursts of light on cancerous tissue.

Since the nineteenth century it has been known that different types of light—sunlight and fractions of it, infrared and ultraviolet—have the power to kill bacteria and neutralise infection. When light is combined with agents that cause photosensitisation this ability is dramatically enhanced. For example, ultraviolet light kills the bacteria Infusorian nassula in nine minutes, but when a photodynamic agent is used as well the time is reduced to ten seconds. Hypericum contains two such photodynamic agents—hypericin and pseudohypericin—found mainly in the red-black oil glands dotted on the surface of the leaves, buds and petals. To be strictly accurate chlorophyll, the molecule present in all green plants and responsible for photosynthesis, should also be listed as a third photodynamic agent. Most attention has, however, been paid to hypericin, for it has a highly significant range of effects within the body. It is clearly the key antiviral constituent within the herb, and has marked photodynamic and anti-cancer activity.

ANTIVIRAL ACTIVITY

Scientists first started to become interested in hypericum as an antiviral agent in the mid-1980s, particularly so when it became apparent that hypericin and pseudohypericin might be effective in treating HIV and AIDS. In view of this it is surprising that there has been far less research into hypericum as an antiviral than as an anti-depressant, although there is now much evidence to show that the herb is a versatile medicine for a wide range of viral infections. What is more, as with its use in depressive illness, it has a very low incidence of side-effects.

Hypericin and viral infections

Viruses, which are hundreds of times smaller than many cells, come in two basic forms:

- Non-enveloped viruses are simple, naked bits of RNA (genetic material); examples include the polio virus and adenoviruses which cause infections such as viral pneumonia.
- Enveloped viruses have a core of RNA surrounded by a fatty (lipid) envelope; examples include influenza and herpes viruses, HIV and hepatitis B and C.

St John's wort and hypericin are thought to have little activity against non-enveloped viruses. They do, however, have specific activity against retroviruses such as HIV, a type of enveloped virus that enters the host cell by merging its 'envelope' with the cell wall, and once within the cell, programmes it to produce more viruses. It achieves this self-production by making a DNA copy of its own RNA, using an enzyme known as *reverse transcriptase*. This DNA copy or code then joins with the DNA in the host cell's nucleus, and the host cell starts to produce the encoded RNA, leading via a number of stages to the replication of the whole virus. Hypericin, and hypericum, appear to block this process of viral replication at a number of key points though the exact details are far from clear:

- It protects *uninfected* cells from infection, by interfering with the virus's ability to 'open up' the cell wall and gain entry. Hypericin works here by binding with the cell membrane.[2, 3] But it also enters into the cell, where
- it inactivates the virus in *infected* cells by blocking release of reverse transcriptase, thus preventing the virus from 'uncoating' itself and initiating the whole sequence that leads to replication of the virus within the cell.[3]

Hypericin's photodynamic activity contributes significantly to both stages, preventing the virus from entering the cell and from 'uncoating' itself, and thereby releasing enzymes essential for it to replicate itself. Though light increases hypericin's antiviral activity, it is still markedly viricidal in the dark. As hypericin is antiviral in both light and dark conditions, it is suspected that more than one mechanism is involved in the process. Early investigations showed that light exposure caused hypericin to transfer energy to nearby oxygen molecules, producing a damaging product called singlet oxygen that is highly toxic to viruses and bacteria. But later experiments showed that hypericin was still toxic even when no nearby oxygen was available. Hypericin may work here by blocking molecules that act as messengers for viral replication in HIV and other viral-infected cells, in particular protein kinase C and protein-kinase tyrosine.[3]

Recent research also shows that when light strikes the hypericin molecule it triggers a chemical reaction called a double proton transfer, which might also be responsible for hypericin's toxic effect against bacteria and viruses. In hypericin, proton transfer reactions occur when a proton, or positively charged hydrogen atom, moves a short distance of less than two angstroms (eight billionths of an inch) between neighbouring oxygen atoms on a molecule.[4] This discovery raises the possibility that hypericin (and hypericum) could be used to treat HIV and AIDS, hepatitis, brain tumours and other diseases.[4] Hypericin's disease-fighting properties are not yet clinically proven, but they are beginning to be evaluated in clinical trials. It has been shown to possess activity against these viruses:

- HIV type 1
- Herpes simplex virus type 1 and type 2
- Para-influenza 3 virus
- Vesicular stomatitis virus[3]

HIV
The antiviral, disease-fighting properties of hypericin (and pseudo-hypericin) are not yet clinically proven, though the processes by which they work are increasingly well understood. Hypericum, and hypericin, have definite potential as treatments for human viral infection but at the present time their effectiveness in practice can only be guessed at.[1] As mentioned earlier, little clinical research using hypericum or hypericin in viral infections has so far been undertaken, though the picture is beginning to change.

Clinical studies
The studies which have taken place with HIV and hypericum or hypericin have been mixed in their results, though recent research is more promising. The most significant work has been under way in Bonn, Germany, for several years. In a poster presented to the International Conference on AIDS in 1993, Drs Steinbeck-Klose and Wernet[5] reported the results of a study involving 18 HIV patients at varying stages of development of the disease. Sixteen

of them had been undergoing treatment for 40 months—that is, until the time of the presentation.

> Clinically, it was noteworthy that only two of these 16 patients encountered an opportunistic infection during the 40 months of observation. The other patients remained clinically stable and are active in work and life . . . *Hypericum perforatum* is presented as a novel effective antiviral substance of broader activity . . . it should be noted that no side-effects have been seen or measured in any of the 16 patients.

It should be stressed that treatment in this study involved two injections per week of hyperforat (a hypericum extract for intravenous use, equivalent to 0.8mg of hypericin) and two tablets of hypericum taken orally three times a day (dose not given). As a consequence, one cannot really draw any firm conclusions about how much the oral use of hypericum is effective for HIV infection.

Two other studies have involved people self-medicating or the simultaneous use of drugs such as AZT. The first, involving 11 patients[6] who were self-medicating with standardised extracts of hypericum, suggests that symptomatic problems such as fatigue, nausea and swollen lymph glands improved quickly, though changes in CD4 cells (the main 'marker' of HIV infection) were slower to occur. However, nine of the 11 reported successful and often dramatic results. In the second study,[7] undertaken over four months, the use of AZT and hypericum combined led to significant falls in CD4 levels, but there was a slight increase in CD4 levels in those taking hypericum alone. In a further study, using hypericin rather than hypericum, presented to the 1991 International Conference on AIDS, 'no early marked anti-HIV activity was found'. There were several reported mild side-effects. Other HIV and AIDS patients have been given synthetic hypericin at very high doses and suffered from rashes and blistering of the skin; but even at this dosage side-effects disappeared on discontinuing treatment. Further clinical trials using synthetic hypericin to treat HIV infection are under way in the USA. In one ongoing trial in New York, patients take up to 20mg of hypericin, in capsule form, on a daily basis.

However, hypericin, whether naturally derived or synthetic, may offer no clear advantage over hypericum, and as a rule hypericum extracts are preferable due to their lower level of side-effects (the buffering effect of other constituents within the plant). A number of researchers now favour a combination of the hypericum extract and hypericin.

An ongoing trial involving 18 AIDS patients given injections of hypericin (1 × 2ml per week) and high doses of hypericum extract (6 × 2 tablets (Jossa) a day) for four to six years was presented at the 1996 International Conference on AIDS.[8] In most patients there was a clear reduction in viral load or level of virus within the blood. In some patients there was an increase in viral load over a three-year period but they did not develop common opportunistic infections such as cytomegalovirus. The scientists concluded that the findings provided strong support for the use of hypericin and its plant-derived form (*Hypericum perforatum*) as a non-toxic and effective long-term antiviral treatment for HIV and AIDS. More trials are under way.

Following this and other trials, it is evident that hypericum extract is a treatment worth considering for HIV infection. Unlike other antiviral drugs it is unlikely to be affected by the development of drug-resistant virus strains, a problem which affects all other antiviral agents. Though the benefits to be gained are not yet clearly established, hypericum's overall safety record when taken long term is strongly in its favour—over 20 million Germans are now thought to have taken standard dose hypericum extracts for more than 12 months. Given that HIV and AIDS patients need to maintain their immune resistance at as high a level as possible, hypericum offers potential long-term benefit with low potential risk. That being said, however, *anyone considering taking hypericum for HIV should always do so only on the basis of professional advice, based on a thorough assessment of all factors involved.*

Herpes virus infections

Herpes viruses are nature's opportunists, causing infection when their host is at his or her weakest. Herpes simplex is the commonest of the six herpes viruses, causing cold stores, mouth ulcers, whitlows, and genital sores. Up to 80 per cent of the population are thought to have had herpes simplex infection at one time or other—often during early childhood. Other common herpes infections include chickenpox and shingles, and glandular fever. Less common herpes infections, such as cytomegalovirus (CMV) which infects the lungs causing pneumonitis, develop only when the immune system is severely compromised. To some degree, though, all herpes infection (other than chickenpox) can be seen as a sign of weakened immune and nervous function.

Although clinical research on herpes infection and hypericum is yet to take place, traditional herbal medicine provides a fairly consistent picture of the herb's use in treating some herpetic problems. In Anglo-American herbal medicine, hypericum is frequently used to treat the nervous and immune depletion that accompanies outbreaks of herpes sores and shingles.[9] Such outbreaks are usually brought on by emotional and physical stress, such as shock, anxiety, or exposure to cold. After an initial infection the virus remains dormant within nerve tissue, emerging to produce symptoms when the immune system is sufficiently weakened. Sharp, sometimes excruciating, nerve pain is all too often the main symptom, occurring where the sores or blisters erupt. Treatment focuses on restoring immune and nervous function, hypericum acting here not simply as an antiviral, but as an analgesic and nerve tonic.[10]

Known with good reason as 'arnica for the nerves', due to its ability to relieve nerve pain in the same way that arnica (*Arnica montana*) relieves the pain of wounds and bruises, hypericum is applied externally as an oil to the sores and at the same time taken internally. Rubbed in gently, the oil will reduce pain though the process may be slow. Indeed, hypericum may not be particularly effective in treating acute attacks, so much as supporting long-term recovery and in the process earning its title of 'nerve restorative'. Probably, the best bet for herpes simplex and shingles is to use hypericum extracts in the medium to long term combined with other treatment that will have a more immediate effect—for example, echinacea (*Echinacea* spp.) internally, with lemon balm (*Melissa officinalis*) and hypericum ointment applied to sores.

Whether hypericum might prove an effective treatment for other herpes infections is not known. Two factors, however, suggest it should be of value in treating glandular fever, caused by the Epstein-Barr virus: the established antiviral activity and a possible liver protective action. Liver function is often abnormal in glandular fever and the liver can become significantly enlarged. Hypericum may well act to support normal liver function (see next section). Certainly, herbalists commonly use hypericum in glandular fever in conjunction with other herbs that support liver or immune function, not least because nervous and physical exhaustion are common features of this illness, which particularly strikes teenagers and students. A further and very sketchy possibility is that hypericum might be valuable in treating or preventing the development of multiple sclerosis (MS). Scientists have linked the human herpes virus-6 (HHV-6) with the onset of MS,[11] although as 90 per cent of the adult American population have the virus and only a few people develop MS it is clearly not the only 'cause' (see chapter 9 for further details). Finally, it is probable that hypericum will be helpful in countering opportunistic infections such as cytomegalovirus, which occur frequently in people with compromised immune systems—perhaps a further reason for its use in HIV and AIDS.

Again, one returns to the herb's truly remarkable range of therapeutic effects which together make it potentially suitable for conditions caused by a weakened immune system. Does it make sense to talk about hypericum as an anti-immune depressant, as well as an anti-depressant? Where immune function is compromised the gentle support provided by hypericum for mood, nervous function, immune resistance and liver function adds up to quite a powerful package.

Hepatitis B and C, and liver protective activity

Although there is no published information on the use of hypericum extracts for hepatitis, a number of medical practitioners in Germany are using relatively high doses of the herb to treat people with hepatitis C virus (HCV). Given that HCV is a retrovirus, and that HCV patients face chronic liver damage in the medium to long term as the viral load increases, hypericum offers a low risk, potentially high benefit treatment for this condition.

There is also preliminary evidence to suggest that hypericum might act to protect the liver itself. Animal studies in China using *Hypericum japonicum*, a species native to China, showed positive results in preventing signs of liver damage, with liver function returning almost to normal after treatment.[12] A further animal study, this time in Turkey and using *Hypericum perforatum*, ended on a strongly affirmative note:

> In conclusion, it is suggested that *H. perforatum* has a protective effect on the liver. Since this plant also exerts antiviral activity, it might be expected that *Hypericum perforatum* and its constituents will be used as potential tools for the treatment of viral hepatitis.[13]

An additional factor in favour of hypericum is that interferon, which can produce severe side-effects and make some patients worse, is the only conventional treatment available. Clearly, evidence for hypericum's effectiveness in HCV is lacking, but the signs are that long-term treatment, well over a year, using about twice the normal dosage of hypericum extract—6 × 300mg a day—produces consistently beneficial results. I have treated two patients with HCV for two years, using hypericum with herbs such as milk thistle (*Silybum marianum*) and echinacea (*Echinacea* spp.), and in both cases their liver function has returned almost to normal and their general health has noticeably improved. Although no one is in a position to say with certainty that long-term treatment with relatively large doses of hypericum is entirely safe, the general view within the medical and herbal world is that potential risks are slight, if any exist at all. Despite this, as with HIV, *self-medication for this condition is ill-advised and cannot be recommended. Liver function and the individual's response to treatment need to be closely monitored by a medical, herbal or naturopathic practitioner.*

* * *

To sum up, hypericum shows real promise as a safe and effective treatment for human retroviral infection, though the clinical evidence for it is simply not there yet. People with chronic retroviral infection, especially HIV and HCV, are quite likely to benefit from taking the extract long term; however, *they should do so only with professional advice and regular monitoring.*

It may also be misleading to think of hypericum as the viral equivalent of an antibiotic (which kills bacteria, not viruses), for although hypericum and hypericin kill viruses very effectively in laboratory conditions, it is not clear that they work effectively in this way within the body. People with HIV and HCV infection treated with hypericum respond only after months of treatment, and nowhere is there any evidence that acute viral conditions such as influenza respond quickly when treatment with hypericum begins. In common with many other herbal medicines, it is likely that hypericum achieves its effects slowly, working with the body's own immune defences and protecting the cell from viral entry.

The entry for hypericum in *Botanical Medicine: A European Professional Perspective* states that the herb 'strengthens the immune system and is particularly indicated for infections that are chronic or recurrent'.[14] Following on this idea, hypericum is perhaps better thought of as an immune 'protector' or 'enhancer' in retroviral infection than as an antiviral, and it is worth recalling that one way it acts as an antiviral is by preventing the cell wall from being breached by the virus. It may genuinely make sense to consider the herb as an anti-immune depressant.

Finally, to return to the theme of light, going out during the day, especially when the sun is out, will increase hypericum's antiviral activity in the body. But one must be careful—sunbathing is definitely not a good idea, and people prone to sunburn should take great care.

CHAPTER 5

Further Uses of Hypericum—Wound and Tissue Healer

A balsam prepared from St John's wort is a most precious remedy for deep wounds, and those that are through the body; for the sinews that are pricked, or any wound made with a venomed weapon.

Gerard (1597)

Hypericum has been prized as a wound-healer or vulnerary for at least 2,500 years, with dozens of references in herbals and pharmacopoeias across Europe attesting to its virtue in healing damaged tissue. Dioscorides (c.AD 40–90), a Greek army surgeon and author of the first major European herbal, *De Materia Medica*, recommended applying hypericum to burns, and external use of the herb has been popular since this time. Uses have included the cleansing of foul wounds with hypericum oil by surgeons in the 'operating theatre',[1] the treatment of ulcers and sores, and internal and surface wounds with infusion or oil. The herb is particularly associated with the treatment of stabs and war wounds—in parts of Spain it is known as *hierba militar*[2]—possibly because the translucent oil glands dotted across the leaves had the look of needle pricks, but equally because the herb leaves blood-coloured stains on the hand when picked or chopped. The seventeenth-century English herbalist Nicholas Culpeper[3] described it as 'a singular wound herb; boiled in wine and drank, it healeth inward hurts or bruises; made into an ointment, it opens obstructions, dissolves swellings, and closes up the lips of wounds.'

69

Here, as is so often the case, scientific research supports the longstanding experience of herbalists. Hypericum extracts, including the oil, exert a strong antimicrobial and astringent activity that counters and prevents infection, tightens damaged tissue, stimulates scab formation and speeds up tissue repair. When hypericum oil was used topically, 'First degree burns healed in 48 hours', states the American Herbal Pharmacopoeia citing a 1975 study, and 'second and third degree burns healed at least three times as rapidly as burns treated with conventional methods.'[4] Dioscorides, practising nearly 2,000 years ago, would not have been surprised!

Hypericum extracts have been shown to inhibit bacteria at dilutions as low as 1:200,000 and are bactericidal at 1:20,000.[5] Extracts have significant activity against a range of bacteria including *Staphylococcus aureus*, *Proteus vulgaris* and *E. coli*,[6] and against the tuberculosis bacillus.[7] It has a slight antifungal[8] and, as discussed in the previous chapter, significant antiviral activity. At the same time hypericum has marked anti-inflammatory action when applied to the skin or taken internally, making it useful in reducing or relieving the heat, swelling and tenderness that develop whenever tissue damage has occurred, for example in sprains, bruises and cuts. Although one would not want surgeons to rely on hypericum oil for the cleansing of wounds today, its antimicrobial/ antiviral, astringent and anti-inflammatory actions together make a formidable combination for the treatment of wounds, bruises, burns and a range of skin lesions including ulcers, whitlows, cold sores and so on. Indeed, hypericum—both infusion and oil—is distinctly *undervalued* as a local wound healer, in spite of the fact that it also seems able to relieve pain, especially nerve pain. A common and important traditional use of the herb is to relieve toothache and aid recovery from tooth extractions, the oil being massaged into the jaw or cheek overlying the affected area.

One might also add that the herb's anti-depressant and tranquillising effects will aid tissue healing where the person concerned has been suffering from long-term stress. Research into people recovering from heart surgery shows that chronic stress impairs the body's ability to heal and self-repair.[9] Hypericum might therefore be of value in aiding recovery from operations in those who have been subject to chronic stress.

Following Culpeper's empirical experience of 350 years ago, simple extracts of the herb taken internally do seem to be effective in stimulating tissue repair. There is evidence to show that hypericum can aid healing of internal lesions such as stomach ulcers, as well as external wounds. In an animal study, hypericum tincture (1:10) was more effective in healing superficial skin wounds, when given internally, than a calendula (*Calendula officinalis*) tincture applied directly to the site of the wound.[10] Hypericum also proved more effective than calendula in stimulating new skin growth. As calendula or marigold is the most widely used natural wound-healer in Europe, used in both herbal medicine and homoeopathy, this comparison gives some insight into the efficacy of hypericum in stimulating tissue repair.

A small-scale study in the USA, involving five healthy human volunteers, examined the healing properties of several medicinal plants including hypericum and calendula.[11] In those taking the extracts the rate of wound-healing was increased on average by 16 per cent. Interestingly, a commonly available ointment, Hyper-cal, for cuts, wounds, abrasions and painful and inflamed skin, combines the two herbs together. Both herbs are also widely used in cosmetics, with hypericum being thought to aid healing in sunburn. A further unexpected use for hypericum has been put forward in post-Chernobyl Russian research on animals. The study suggests that hypericum may have a protective activity against radiation— the bone marrow and small intestine of mice, given sufficient levels of an infusion of hypericum, were protected against X-ray induced damage.[12]

Hypericum's ability to heal wounds, stimulate tissue repair and prevent infection clearly results from the combined action of a number of constituents—notably the proanthocyanidins; flavonoids; essential oil; hypericin and pseudohypericin; and ad/hyperforin. All contribute to the wound-healing activity while hypericin and hyperforin are particularly important for the broad spectrum antibiotic activity of the herb.

Hypericum—particularly the oil, is therefore a valuable and underused treatment for topical problems such as burns, bruises, cuts, abrasions, tooth extractions and haemorrhoids. Herpes sores and blisters, and whitlows, may also respond well to topical treatment. Its safety also makes it a very useful household remedy for minor burns and wounds in general. See chapter 8 for preparation and application of hypericum oil.

Stomach ulcers, irritable bowel and haemorrhoids

In the same way that hypericum promotes wound-healing on the surface of the body, it can be used to encourage the repair of part of our internal 'skin', specifically the lining of the stomach. Hypericum oil has been used for centuries, notably in Germany, to treat inflammatory problems and ulcers in the stomach. Standard recommended treatment is to take one teaspoon of hypericum oil on an empty stomach morning and night.[13] Treatment needs to be continued for several months, and is best supplemented by other approaches—chamomile tea, change in diet and so on. It is probable that the tincture and infusion, as well as the oil, will be helpful. In a trial already discussed (see 'Addictions', p. 56), alcoholics suffering from depression and gastritis and/or stomach ulcers took regular infusions of hypericum and received psychotherapy: treatment proved effective after two months.[14] In another study, on animals, both hypericum oil and a methanolic extract were found to be effective in healing stomach ulcers.[15]

Another less serious though far more common problem, which could respond well to hypericum in combination with herbs such as peppermint (*Mentha piperita*), is irritable bowel syndrome (IBS). IBS is closely linked to depression, though whether depression causes the problem, or the discomforting experience of IBS—bloating, abdominal pains, urgency, constipation and diarrhoea—causes depression is unclear. With marked astringent and anti-inflammatory activity, hypericum can reduce diarrhoea and irritability within the gut, where it will also encourage repair of the gut wall. As an antimicrobial it may possibly have some effect on gut flora (bacteria within the gut), and the herb has been shown to slow down the rate of peristalsis (muscular contraction of the gut wall). Indeed, this bowel-slowing effect was considered so effective in Russian research published in 1979, that it was suggested that hypericum might be used to slow down the colon for X-ray study.[16] This action on the gut could also be responsible for some of the side-effects linked with hypericum intake. A recent report described the case of a 67-year-old diabetic woman diagnosed as suffering from adynamic ileus (loss of movement of the small intestine), who experienced abdominal distension, bloating, discomfort and constipation. All symptoms slowly eased and cleared within a week of stopping hypericum.[17] Perhaps, in people with 'hyperdynamic' intestinal function such as IBS, hypericum at relatively high dosage might prove therapeutically useful.

'External' haemorrhoids can be treated topically with hypericum oil, which can also be administered as an overnight retention enema for painful and inflamed internal haemorrhoids, and for inflammatory problems within the colon.[13]

Anti-inflammatory action

Turning from the herb's use in local healing—wounds, burns, stomach inflammation and so on, there is significant potential to use hypericum to treat inflammatory conditions which affect the body as a whole. In fact medical herbalists and naturopaths have used hypericum for systemic inflammation for many years, especially in auto-immune disease where the body's immune system is effectively attacking itself.

Detailed study of the microcellular processes involved in inflammation and viral infection have led to the recognition that hypericum's (and hypericin) activity as an anti-inflammatory, antiviral and anti-tumour remedy all appear to be closely linked to its ability to block protein kinase C (PKC) release from the cell wall.[18] PKC plays a major role in intracellular communication—it is a 'signal transductor', and controls a range of cellular activity including cell proliferation and differentiation. It is involved in initiating an inflammatory response, and may have a key role in both viral replication and in the development of cancer (looked at in more detail in the following section). Hypericin's ability to block release by receptors in the cell wall of signal transductors such as PKC and tyrosine kinase, and to protect the cell membrane from viral infection, is further evidence that it has immense therapeutic potential.

Hypericum and hypericin also inhibit the release from white blood cells of arachidonic acid, and its metabolite leukotriene B4— both of which stimulate inflammation.[19] They also block release of interleukin -1α, a potent cytokine that stimulates inflammation and fever, triggers a generalised immune response[19] and may be involved in increased CRH release within the brain, leading in turn to raised cortisol levels and the onset of depression. Interestingly, interleukin -1α was also inhibited by a hypericum extract from which hypericin had been removed, raising the question of just how much hypericin is central to hypericum's anti-inflammatory activity.[19] Hypericum has also been shown *in vitro* to cause a 'massive suppression' of interleukin-6 (IL-6) release,[20] a cytokine which along with IL-1 is closely linked to rheumatoid arthritis.

Given this significant group of anti-inflammatory mechanisms, one can speculate that hypericum will be useful in preventing tissue damage in systemic inflammatory illnesses such as Crohn's disease and rheumatoid arthritis. There has, however, been no clinical research in this area, and there is limited research into the herb's anti-inflammatory activity in general. Reporting the results of an animal study, a paper in the *British Homoeopathic Journal*[21] concluded that there was no statistical difference between hypericum tincture and hydrocortisone in relieving arthritic inflammation. Interestingly, the researchers found that at relatively low doses (0.25ml/100g body weight) the anti-inflammatory effect was 48 per cent, while at double the dose anti-inflammatory activity fell to 32 per cent. Tantalisingly, that appears to be the only published study on hypericum as an anti-inflammatory.

Nonetheless, medical herbalists commonly use hypericum for systemic inflammatory disorders such as rheumatoid arthritis (RA), and it is worthwhile considering the ways in which the herb might influence such disorders. RA may have a viral cause, and its onset is certainly linked to both stress and digestive disturbance. It typically produces inflammation affecting peripheral joints such as the hands and feet, and can involve a very broad range of other symptoms including anaemia, and heart and chest problems. There is also a strong association of RA and depression,[22] and hypericum may help in such auto-immune conditions on a number of levels:

- countering joint and muscle inflammation and encouraging repair of damaged tissue;
- countering viral triggers that may lie behind the disordered immune response causing the condition;
- strengthening the integrity of the gut wall: 'leaky' gut, which involves a) damage to the inner lining of the gut wall e.g. from aspirin and similar medicines, and b) the absorption of allergenic and toxic material, is linked to auto-immune conditions;
- relieving pain (topical use mainly);
- easing depression and nervous exhaustion, which commonly occurs with RA; relieving anxiety and generally encouraging a more positive mood.

As a medical herbalist I would not want to rely solely on hypericum to treat RA—it would not make sense. But it certainly figures well up my list of preferred herbs for this condition, and deserves further investigation.

Anti-cancer

Research into hypericum's potential as an anti-cancer treatment is still in its early stages, with hypericin being actively studied for use as an anti-cancer drug. Current treatments for cancer tend to be indiscriminate in their action, affecting healthy and cancerous tissue alike, and often producing severe side-effects. For medical researchers the exciting possibility is that hypericin can be precisely targeted to destroy cancer cells, leaving healthy ones unaffected. Utilising hypericin's light-sensitive activity, researchers are trying to 'switch on' the molecule within targeted cancerous cells, by using very short bursts of laser light. The theory is that light causes the molecule to undergo two proton transfer reactions at the same time, one on either side of the molecule. Hypericin can of course produce photosensitisation at high dosage, but the dose required for effective anti-cancer and antiviral activity appears to be below the level where skin sensitisation develops.

Hypericin exerts an anti-cancer and anti-tumour effect via a number of other pathways, some of which have already been discussed in earlier sections. They include:

- Inhibition of enzymes such as protein kinase C, tyrosine kinase and epidermal growth factor, which influence cell proliferation and differentiation. These molecules, via a complex cascade of actions, can act as tumour growth promoters. There is also an effect inducing programmed cell death (apoptosis) which encourages cell 'suicide' in what might otherwise become cancerous cells.[23]
- Inhibition of the enzyme succonidase in mitochondria (cellular 'power plants'), involved in cancerous changes in cells. This effect is six times stronger in the presence of light.[18]
- Other light-dependent/photodynamic activity producing a direct effect on tumour cells, including 'singlet oxygen', which causes free radical damage within viruses and cancer cells, as well as the 'double proton transfer' reaction, which might make it effective in cancers such as glioblastoma, a highly malignant brain tumour.[24]
- Direct antiviral activity against viruses which cause leukaemia.[18]
- Cytotoxic activity against mouse breast cancer cells. Studies have shown hypericin to be equal to or more effective than Tamoxifen, the standard treatment for breast cancer.[18]

This is quite a list, and one that explains why scientists are so interested in hypericin as a future cancer treatment. Research is under way in a number of centres in the USA, including the US Department of Energy's Brookhaven National Laboratory in

Upton, NY, and is being sponsored by several pharmaceutical and biotechnology companies. At UCLA research is under way into hypericin as a treatment for skin cancers. It is, however, worthwhile distinguishing between hypericin's (and to some extent hypericum's) potential role as a *treatment* for cancer, and hypericum's role in *preventing* cancer, resulting from the combined effect of many of its constituents—hypericin, pseudohypericin, proanthocyanidins, flavonoids and others. While hypericin, and to a lesser extent pseudohypericin, hold out promise as effective anti-cancer agents, it seems more or less self-evident that hypericum, in common with the many other plants that have antioxidant activity (both foods and medicines), has a direct preventative role in cancer, preventing free radical damage including scavenging superoxide anions and inhibiting lipid peroxidation. At present, hypericum's preventative role is probably the one that has the most direct relevance, and all those taking the herb long term are likely to benefit from this effect.

Heart and circulation
Although hypericum has been used in Italy to treat low blood pressure,[6] no other evidence exists to suggest that the herb has been valued in the past for heart or circulatory problems. With the discovery that the plant contains high levels of proanthocyanidins (approximately 12 per cent), which protect and strengthen the cardiovascular system and have a vasodilatory action on arteries and capillaries, hypericum clearly has beneficial effects on the heart and circulation. Moreover, the plant and its procyanidins are strongly antioxidant and have a protective activity against free-radical damage. Russian research published in 1998 demonstrated that, of the seven herbs evaluated, hypericum had the greatest antioxidant activity.[25] Procyanidins found at high levels in hawthorn (*Crataegus* spp.), a native European tree, are largely responsible for its established medicinal use in cardiovascular disease—countering arteriosclerosis, supporting heart function, and increasing blood flow to the heart via dilation of the coronary arteries. Isolated procyanidins from hypericum act *in vitro* in a more or

less identical manner to those found in hawthorn,[26] and appear to block biochemical processes (phosphodiesterase and/or angiotensin converting enzyme),[27] which cause arterial spasm and make the heart work harder. In clinical trials, hawthorn has been shown to markedly improve the working capacity of the heart in people with mild chronic heart failure, and to reduce heart rate and systolic blood pressure.[28] Indeed, hawthorn is considered a 'heart protector', being widely used as a medicine in Germany for angina, coronary artery disease and high blood pressure.

Quite reasonably, one can deduce from all this that hypericum, too, positively influences cardiovascular function, in particular supporting the heart when under stress—even though precise evidence is lacking. The one trial that examined hypericum's cardiovascular effects did so in the context of its use as an anti-depressant. Hypericum extract (1800mg) and imipramine (a tricyclic anti-depressant) were compared for their impact on the heart function of 209 patients suffering from depression. After six weeks those taking imipramine showed increased abnormalities in heart function, especially in heart conductivity, while those taking hypericum extract showed a significant reduction in such pathological findings. The researchers noted that hypericum extract should be preferred to tricyclic anti-depressants for patients who are elderly or suffer from heart disorders.[29]

Other constituents in hypericum also have a positive effect on the circulation—hypericin has been reported to increase capillary circulation[30]—but perhaps, following Paracelsus, we should look at the herb more as a treatment for 'downheartedness', as a remedy for the emotional heart, than for problems of the physical heart.

The heart has always been seen as the seat of the emotions, and many heart disorders, for example angina and sudden-onset heart failure, have a strong stress-related element. Furthermore, disordered serotonin levels have been implicated in sudden cardiac death. Most people instinctively recognise that severe emotional shock damages the heart, and know that it is possible literally to die of a 'broken heart'. Maybe hypericum is best understood as a herb that helps to heal the wounds of grief and hopelessness that follow loss or bereavement, while quietly providing physiological support to the physical functioning of the heart. Working here primarily as an anti-depressant and anti-anxiety remedy, it will at the same time aid blood flow through the coronary arteries, open up the arteries and capillaries (thus lightening the load on a stressed heart), and encourage regular heart function. Though there are better herbal medicines for the heart and circulation, hypericum's value in supporting healthy cardiovascular function should not be underestimated.

CHAPTER 6

St John's Wort in History

St John's wort, St John's wort,
My envy whosoever has thee, '
I will pluck thee with my right hand,
I will preserve thee with my left hand,
Whoso findeth thee in the cattlefold,
Shall never be without kine [cattle].

A Gaelic incantation collected from the
Hebrides (Scotland) by Alexander Carmichael (1900)

In the developed world where mainstream medical care is high-tech and based on chemical drug treatment, it can come as a shock to realise that around 80 per cent of the world rely to this day on plant medicines when they fall ill. Even in developed countries about 25 per cent of all medicines come from medicinal plants, and this figure does not include the growing use of herbal medicines in Western societies. A saying attributed to Aesculapius, a Greek deity who is supposed to have lived in the twelfth century BC, neatly sums up humanity's debt to medicinal plants—*first the word, then the herb, lastly the knife.* Whenever love, friendship or wise counsel have proved unable to heal illness, people's first recourse has been to medicinal herbs. By and large it still is, and seen from this perspective, our growing reliance on chemical medicines may one day be seen as an historical aberration.

If even today the greater part of the world relies on medicinal plants for medicine, then in the past reliance must have been almost total. Living much closer to nature than we do today, our ancestors were acute observers of plant and animal life, and had a shrewd understanding of how most plants could be used as foods and medicines. We in Europe can only guess at the ancient understanding and use of medicinal plants before the earliest written records, but the experience of ethnobotanists working with native peoples over the last two decades, for example in the Amazon region,[1] would suggest that their understanding was sophisticated and subtle, and involved a deep knowledge of plant lore—botany and herbal medicine. Plants that most of us would see as identical are often carefully distinguished from each other in such pre-literate societies, though little distinction is made between a plant's magical and mythical powers and its medicinal or pharmacological activity: magic and medicine are always intimately entwined, even today, in the era of Viagra and organ transplants! Medicine in this broad sense of the word is the power to influence one's environment, specifically the internal environment of the body. Medicinal plants such as St John's wort were strong medicine, because of their visible but unaccountable power to heal wounds, counter infection and restore good health.

MAGIC AND FOLK MEDICINE

Ancient civilisations around the world in China, Egypt, India, Mexico and elsewhere had an acute awareness of the passage of the sun, moon and stars 'around' the earth. By closely observing the sun and moon—and the inherent rhythms that they give to all life on our planet—changes in the seasons and tides could be confidently predicted and a 'divine' order placed on the world. By extension, medicinally-active plants that flowered or fruited at specific times within these cycles, especially at the winter and summer solstices, had great magical power. Their therapeutic virtues were drawn from the sun—the literal source of life on earth—and could offer protection against illness and against ills in general. St John's wort's burst of yellow flowers around the time of the summer solstice signified the plant's unusual powers and the herb was used traditionally throughout Europe as a herb of light, protecting against and banishing the powers of darkness and gloom. The herb's yellow-gold flowers of course increased its correspondence with the sun, encouraging the weaving of yet more magical charms into the protective fabric of its sun-warmed foliage.

St John's wort is one of the foremost European herbs linked to the summer solstice, perhaps representing the sun at the peak of its powers at the point of decline. Mistletoe, in its link with the winter solstice and the gradual rebirth of the sun that follows, had greater ritual significance—there is more myth and folklore attached to the 'Golden Bough', as Virgil called mistletoe in his Latin epic the *Aeniad*, than almost any other European plant. Commonly acknowledged as the sacred herb of the Druids, its magical uses have survived to this day in Christmas festivities, while its medicinal uses are being intensively investigated. In contrast, hypericum fell into disrepute as both a magical and a medicinal plant in the nineteenth century, its reappraisal as a medicine beginning only about 20 years ago.

It is very probable that St John's wort was used at the great midsummer festival that was celebrated in pre-Christian Britain and Europe,[2, 3] in much the same way that mistletoe was used in celebrations at the winter solstice. One part of the midsummer festivities was the lighting of bonfires on which ceremonial herbs, usually yellow-flowered, were burnt or smoked over the fires. St John's wort was one of the main plants used, but others included vervain (*Verbena officinalis*), tormentil (*Potentilla erecta*) and cinquefoil (*Potentilla reptans*). No precise knowledge exists, however, and one can only surmise from the herb's botanical name— derived from the Greek words *hyper* and *eikon*, meaning 'over' and 'icon' as in 'above an apparition'[4]—that it has always been used to ward off evil spirits. One tradition states that St John's wort is *Fuga Daemonum*, the plant which the ancient Greeks believed had the power of driving away demons.[2] A German name for the plant is *Hexenkraut* (witches' or magic herb).

British folk traditions also attest to this view, reflecting the ancient belief that midsummer is a time when evil forces are particularly active. In Wales the herb was known as *Y Fendigedig* or 'the blessed'[5] and in many parts of the country a sprig was placed on the doors of houses to free them from evil spirits. Also in Wales, a root of St John's wort dug at midnight on St John's Eve (24 June) was believed capable of driving out devils and witches,[2] while at St Cleer in Cornwall, wreaths of St John's wort were hung around the village to banish witches.

Writing somewhat sceptically in 1777, J. Lightfoot noted:

> the superstitious in Scotland carry this plant about with them as a charm against dire effects of witchcraft and enchantment. They also cure, or fancy they cure, their ropey milk, which they suppose to be under some malignant influence, by putting this herb into it and milking afresh upon it.[6]

Hypericum has not always been used for 'good' magical purposes. Reginald Scot in *The discoverie of Witchcraft* (1584)[3] gives instructions for raising the ghost of a hanged man with a hazel wand, an owl's head and a bundle of St John's wort!

From early Christian times onwards the herb has been associated with St John the Baptist. St Columba, the early Celtic saint who is reputed to have had a great affection for St John the Baptist, is said to have always carried the herb in his armpit and one of its Gaelic names is *achlasan Chalium-chille*, meaning literally the 'armpit package of Columba'.[2]

St John's wort and the doctrine of signatures

Paracelsus (1493–1541), the famous Swiss chemist, doctor and rebellious spirit, considered St John's wort to be a supreme example of the doctrine of signatures, the theory that God had placed a sign in every plant indicating its medicinal use. One had only to look for the sign and its medicinal use would become clear. For Paracelsus 'the holes in the leaves [of St John's wort] mean that this herb helps all inner and outer orifices of the skin ... the blooms rot in the form of blood, a sign that it is good for wounds and should be used where flesh has to be treated.'[7] By way of contrast, a rural English view had it that the holes in the leaves were made by witches out of spite for its (to them) 'inconvenient virtues'.[5] Nonetheless, Paracelsus' interpretation fits

St John's wort particularly well, for on picking or crushing the flowering tops of the plant one's hands are quickly covered in dark red bloodlike stains—caused by hypericins released from within the red-black oil glands. With such a graphically visual sign it is hardly surprising that St John's wort has always been considered a wound herb.

Other authors such as the seventeenth-century English herbalist John Coles have followed Paracelsus in this reading of St John's wort, though few have been as fulsome in their praise of its medicinal uses—'its virtue is beyond all description, how great it truly is and what can be achieved with it . . . it is not possible that any better remedy for wounds will be found in any country.'[8]

CLASSICAL USES OF HYPERICUM

Hypericum was clearly used as a medicine in ancient Greece, though there is confusion about which species were actually employed. Hippocrates is thought to have used *Hypericum coris* as a cooling and anti-inflammatory remedy,[8] and according to one authority in the later Hippocratic school hypericum oil was used for the treatment of depression.[9] The Greek surgeon Dioscorides, in his herbal *De Materia Medica*, lists four species of hypericum, which he recommends for the relief of sciatica, to cleanse the bile ducts, and topically to heal burns. Some species are recommended as diuretics and to stimulate menstruation, and the seeds, drunk for 40 days, could be used to treat chronic recurrent fevers, possibly including malaria.[4, 10]

Pliny the Elder, a Roman author writing at the same time as Dioscorides but lacking his medical knowledge, simply recommends the herb against the bites of poisonous reptiles.[11] Galen, physician to the Roman Emperor Marcus Aurelius, and the ancient world's most prolific medical author, considered hypericum to have hot and dry qualities,[4] useful therefore for correcting or banishing an excess of moist and cold humours, and temperamentally linked to problems related to the brain and to winter. His views on hypericum, as in all other aspects of medicine, were to prove decisive in European medicine for the following 1,400 years,[12] until the new scientific spirit of enquiry took off during the Renaissance.

1450–1800

It is hard to write about hypericum without returning time and again to Paracelsus, for his writing on this herb, as on other subjects, is always provocative. In particular, his enthusiastic belief in hypericum's therapeutic powers—'God has given to Perforatum (St John's wort) the strength to chase the ghosts of nature, also worms, and wounds and bone fractures, and all downheartedness . . . it is truly a universal medicine beyond mankind's creation'[13]— has undoubtedly been one reason why, five centuries later, researchers in Germany began to look into hypericum's potential role as an anti-depressant. Earlier authorities affirmed the use of the plant for problems affecting the nerves, but Paracelsus went much farther in stressing its value in treating depressive states.

In fiercely championing the value of local native medicinal plants such as hypericum in favour of the exotic and expensive imported medicinal plants so commonly prescribed in the sixteenth to eighteenth centuries,[14] Paracelsus also helped to maintain interest in native European plants within the medical profession. His influence on European medicine has been profound and his ideas were later to influence unorthodox medical practitioners including Christian Hahnemann, the founder of homoeopathy, and Father Sebastian Kneipp, one of the major figures in nineteenth-century German naturopathy.

Many of the herbals printed in Europe in the sixteenth and seventeenth centuries, whether in German, French, Italian or English, gave similar information, often repeating the indications given by Dioscorides, Galen and the Arabian physician, Avicenna. Both Hieronymus Bock and Matthiolus, who produced two of the great herbals of the time, include wound-healing, haemostatic (stopping bleeding), diuretic, emmenagogue (stimulating menstruation) and antimalarial activity.[15] For hypericum this repetition did not matter too much for its wound-healing properties were agreed on by all—university-educated physicians, herbalists, and 'cunning' men and women alike—the latter probably providing most medical care outside the main cities.

Hypericum oil was a popular wound remedy and was included in the first London Pharmacopoeia (1616) as *Oleum Hyperici*.[4] Many herbals gave recipes for its preparation, typically infusing the flowering tops in olive oil in a clear glass jar, and leaving it in the sunlight for some weeks. John Gerard gives more complex instructions for a recipe that includes white wine and turpentine.[16] Significantly, he recommends that the process be repeated using a second quantity of herb to produce an oil with sufficient strength. The mid-nineteenth century English *Our Useful Wild Flowers* notes that herbalists still sell the steeped oil of hypericum for use as a vulnerary,[5] and this use of the herb continued through Europe and in Russia, where it has always been an important medicinal plant.

Although the astrological view of the herb really only figured during the two hundred years or so when astrology was in vogue in western Europe (roughly 1480–1680), it is interesting to note that Culpeper describes it as 'under the celestial sign Leo, and the dominion of the Sun'.[17] Burton recommended that it be picked 'on a Friday in the hour of Jupiter'.[5] Paracelsus, however, must have the last word. He states that:

> if one wants to use Perforatum against the phantasmas of which I earlier spoke, gather it according to the celestial orbit. This is so that its influence can be also against those ghosts mostly in Mars, Jupiter, and Venus, and by no means according to the Moon, but contrary to it. Also not in the afternoon or at night but in the Sun's rising.[13]

NINETEENTH-CENTURY USAGE

Amongst herbalists, and in rural areas where country traditions remained firmly rooted, hypericum continued to be used in the nineteenth century as a remedy for wounds, sciatica, urinary and bile duct problems and nervous states. As a general rule, however, it was seen as meriting little attention as a medicine, perhaps being of economic significance as a red dye,[5] for hypericin had been isolated from the herb in 1830 by the German chemist, Buchner.[18] 'Nowadays both the herb and its properties are alike forgotten,' lamented Father Kneipp.[19] In fact, with the emergence in Germany and the USA of new unorthodox forms of medical practice—homoeopathy and naturopathy in particular—traditional herbal practices were being reassessed, and this led in time to a re-evaluation of hypericum.

Kneipp himself wrote that the herb had particular influence upon the liver, might help to relieve headaches, and to resolve bedwetting in children. This latter indication reflected German folk medicine, in which hypericum was frequently used for bedwetting, as well as to encourage menstruation when a period was 'stuck' or absent, for uterine problems, and for bronchial catarrh.[15] Hypericum oil, rather than the herb itself, continued to be used for burns and scalds within both mainstream and naturopathic medicine, instructions for its preparation being included in the 1847 Pharmacopoeia Wirtenbergica.[18]

From a completely different Anglo-American background, John Skelton in his *Family Medical Adviser* (1873)[20] recommended hypericum, taken as an infusion, for diarrhoea, inflammation of the bowels, obstruction of urine and hysterical complaints. An infusion of St John's wort, peppermint (*Mentha piperita*) and cayenne (*Capsicum annuum*) is recommended for measles.

Christian Hahneman used herbs such as arnica (*Arnica montana*) and hypericum both as true homoeopathic medicines—diluted to extremely low doses and taken internally, and as herbal medicines—at normal dose applied as lotions, tinctures or ointments to the skin. The homoeopathic understanding of hypericum drew heavily on past traditional usage, and in due course influenced and broadened views of the herb, for example, amongst naturopaths in Germany and medical herbalists of the North American Eclectic movement. A contemporary list of homoeopathic indications for the herb carries more than echoes of its traditional use in Western herbal medicine:

> The great remedy for injuries to nerves, especially of the fingers, toes and nails . . . punctured or penetrating wounds . . . relieves pain after operations . . . has an important action on the rectum, haemorrhoids . . . injured nerves from bites of animals . . . lacerations . . . injury to the brain or spinal cord . . . the Arnica of the nerves . . . melancholy, brain fag and neurasthenia . . . complaints from fright . . . vertigo . . . neuritis, tingling and burning pain . . . hyperhidrosis [excessive sweating] and sweating of scalp . . . eczema of hands and face . . . herpes zoster [shingles].[21]

Though abbreviated, this list represents a fairly comprehensive summary of the herb's use over the last 2,000 years or so! Although such a broad sweep perspective suits the purposes of homoeopathy, within herbal medicine or phytotherapy, the challenge in the twentieth century has been to establish a sharper focus, identifying the core medicinal activity of the plant. The herb can then be used with a new degree of precision, with confidence in its therapeutic powers reaffirmed.

CHAPTER 7

St John's Wort in Western Herbal Medicine

The wisdom of the empiricist always precedes the scientist.
Majid Ali, *What lions know about stress*, 1997

From the disconcertingly varied historical uses of the herb detailed in the last chapter, the wheel this century has turned full circle. The British Herbal Pharmacopoeia (1983)[1] describes hypericum rather sparsely as a sedative and astringent, with analgesic and antiseptic activity when applied topically. Descriptions in more recent pharmacopoeias do not necessarily provide any more detail—the detail has just changed or in some cases shrunk. The article or monograph on hypericum published by the European Scientific Cooperative for Phytotherapy (1996),[2] more or less the official European Union view of the herb, describes it as indicated for 'mild to moderate depressive states . . . restlessness, anxiety and irritability'. Over the thirteen years between these two authoritative texts, hypericum has become scientifically accepted as an anti-depressant with a huge body of research to back it up. Unfortunately, as we shall see, in the process it appears to have lost all its other activities! A good balance seems to have been struck in the first monograph of the American Herbal Pharmacopoeia (1997) on St John's wort,[3] where the herb is listed for internal use as an 'anti-depressant and wound-healing agent . . . anti-inflammatory, antiviral, astringent, cardiotonic and sedative'; and for external use as an 'analgesic, anti-inflammatory, antimicrobial and vulnerary'.

89

Hypericum has become something of a trail-blazer for herbal medicine, challenging the predominant twentieth-century view that herbal medicines are either too inactive to have medicinal value or too toxic to consider using. In the USA in particular there are signs that awareness of hypericum's value as a medicine, and its remarkable safety record, are leading to a wholesale re-evaluation of the potential of botanical medicines. Ironically, one consequence of this success is that the herb's value in treating depression has come to overshadow its many other therapeutic uses. Hypericum has become known as the herbal anti-depressant (implying that no other herbs with anti-depressant activity exist), and its complex multi-faceted activity as a medicine, based on the observation and experience of generations of herbal and medical practitioners, and enriched by recent research, has been largely ignored.

Throughout this century in herbal medicine, in countries as far apart as Canada, Portugal, Romania, Russia and Australia, hypericum has had consistent use in treating problems related to:

- nervous exhaustion, nerve damage and nerve pain;
- affective and stress-related disorders—anxiety and depression;
- menopausal, and in some traditions, menstrual problems;
- wounds, ulcers and tissue damage in general—internal and local use;
- gastro-intestinal disorders such as stomach ulcers;
- liver and bile duct problems;
- urinary disorders including bedwetting;
- inflammatory conditions.

Not all these uses are common to all parts of the world where *Hypericum perforatum* is used, but there is much overlap and these headings represent the core usage of the herb in Western herbal medicine during the twentieth century—many of course having carried through from the nineteenth century and before.

ST JOHN'S WORT IN WESTERN HERBAL MEDICINE

HYPERICUM AS A 'NERVINE'

King's *American Dispensatory*,[4] a key work based on detailed clinical observation in practice published in 1898, recommends hypericum for suppression of the urine, chronic urinary affections, diarrhoea, dysentery, worms, jaundice and nervous affections with depression, amongst other conditions. Furthermore, hypericum 'has undoubted powers over the nervous system, particularly the spinal cord . . . and is used in injuries of the spine.' Reflecting this range of uses, American, Australasian and British herbalists have mainly used hypericum as a wound-healer, for problems of the urinary and digestive systems, and as a nervine—having a restorative and tonic or relaxant effect on the nervous system.

The idea of a 'nervine' brings together and integrates the wide range of actions, both restorative and tonic, that hypericum and other similar medicinal plants such as vervain have on neuroendocrine function. Nervine herbs provide support for the battered nervous and endocrine systems of people suffering from nervous exhaustion, depression, nerve damage, long-term emotional stress, anxiety, and the like. Such herbs are highly prized by medical herbalists—the herbal practitioners of the English-speaking world—for each patient's overall state of mental, emotional and physiological health is assessed, and nervine herbs are frequently called for. In our time, with ever-growing levels of emotional and mental stress, related perhaps to the breakdown of extended family and community ties, and to environmental pollution and degradation, people more and more need remedies that can support tired or 'burnt-out' nervous systems. Nervines such as hypericum provide at least a partial answer, because they are neither excessively stimulant nor excessively sedative. In fact, the experience of medical herbalists is that nervine remedies tend to normalise mental and emotional state, suggesting that hypericum works on a continuum—acting as a sedative and relaxing those who are anxious and overactive, acting as a stimulant and tonic to whose who are depressed and nervously exhausted. The research to date, examined earlier in this book, would certainly support such a view.

As a nervine, hypericum is usually prescribed along with three or four other herbs that reflect the individual needs of the patient. For example, a 53-year-old man with nervous exhaustion, anxiety, migraines and a stomach ulcer could be given just hypericum, for it will help each of these problems. However, he is likely to do better if herbs such as liquorice (*Glycyrrhiza glabra*), ginkgo (*Ginkgo biloba*), valerian (*Valeriana officinalis*) and chamomile (*Chamomilla recutita*), all strongly indicated, are included in the prescription. From an holistic perspective, hypericum will 'earn its place' in a prescription for chronic ill health of almost any kind, even where nervous exhaustion or depression is not the main problem. The background restorative activity that hypericum exerts on neuro-endocrine-immune function—on serotonin, CRH, cortisol levels and so on—will positively influence the body's physiological capacity to self-heal, while simultaneously encouraging a more positive mental and emotional attitude in the patient.

Hypericum's analgesic activity should not be forgotten, for it has frequently been used to treat damaged nerves and nerve pain—classically in sciatica, where pressure on the sciatic nerve in the lumbar back causes searing pains to run down the path of the nerve from the back and inside leg to the foot. Equally, hypericum has been prescribed to support people with nervous exhaustion and depression resulting from long-term pain. Priest and Priest, British herbalists writing in 1982, concisely summarise the Anglo-American view of the herb as a nervine, listing its uses as 'Painful injuries to sacral spine and coccyx. Traumatic shock. Haemorrhoids with pain/bleeding. Facial neuralgia after dental extractions, toothache. Neurasthenia [nervous exhaustion], chorea [restless writhing movements] and depression.'[5]

Toothache and dental extractions are definitely helped by hypericum in my experience (personal, and with my patients), and the oil massaged into the cheek overlying the problem or into the gum itself will often bring relief and stop bleeding.

While the nervine, 'nerve-nourishing' aspect of hypericum may be the prime focus of American, Australian and British herbalism, the herb has been used commonly for many of the other areas listed above—for example, as an anti-inflammatory for rheumatoid arthritis, and for urinary problems including incontinence and bedwetting.

European usage

In Germany, the influence of Paracelsus has been stronger than elsewhere, despite the 450 years that have elapsed since he died. His view that hypericum was a God-given panacea, with the ability 'to chase away the ghosts of nature, also worms, and to heal wounds and bone fractures, and all down-heartedness' has perhaps been a factor encouraging reappraisal of the herb. Certainly, other than in naturopathic medicine and traditional folk usage, hypericum's use as a medicine had all but ceased in Germany.

Starting from the understanding that hypericum acted as a sedative, phytotherapists, pharmacologists and herbal manufacturers began researching the herb in the 1940s. Slowly evidence of the herb's efficacy as an anti-depressant and wound-healing agent accumulated, with researchers in 1979 listing depressive illness, migraine and psychosomatic symptoms, and bedwetting in children, as hypericum's main uses.[6] By the late 1980s research began literally to snowball. As the evidence has mounted, so hypericum's use has grown by leaps and bounds. An estimated 20 million people in Germany have taken the herb for one year or more, and many, many more have taken it across the world. This massive 'turnaround' over the space of 50 years is due in no small part to the determination and dedication of that small band of German phytotherapists and researchers who believed in the herb's medicinal potential. They should be thanked for bringing a largely overlooked herb 'back to life', for changing the way people regard botanical medicines, and above all for making a safe and effective treatment available for everyone suffering from depressive illness.

As I mentioned in chapter 1, herbal medicine, or phytotherapy as it is called in Europe, is different in Germany. Over 80 per cent of German GPs prescribe herbal medicines, and in 1993 the herbal medicine market in Germany accounted for 50 per cent of the global market in economic terms.[7] In Germany, in contrast to every other Western country, herbal medicines, with their low level of side-effects, are often used as front line treatment for chronic ill health. If the appropriate herbal medicine fails to be effective then conventional chemical medicines will be prescribed. This approach may not be particularly holistic, but as a result a number of medicinal plants, hypericum included, are now the primary form of treatment for conditions as varied as varicose veins, enlarged prostate, insomnia and poor memory. Hypericum itself is widely used for a range of conditions that includes seasonal and other affective disorders, 'burn-out', migraine and chronic headaches, epilepsy, menopausal problems, hepatitis C, stomach ulcers, wounds; and in children, for concentration problems, speech disorders and bedwetting.

In many other European countries, the lead set by Germany has directly influenced the medicinal use of the herb, although older, more traditional, perspectives of the herb continue. For example, the famed Swiss naturopath, Alfred Vogel, who founded the Bioforce herbal manufacturing company, considers hypericum to have greater effect than ginkgo in improving circulation to the capillaries and skin.[8] He also combines hypericum with lemon balm (*Melissa officinalis*) and hops (*Humulus lupulus*) for nervous complaints. In France, following more than ten years' study by H. Leclerc[9] into topical applications of the herb, it has chiefly been used as a local remedy, for itchy, chapped and bruised skin; for burns including sunburn; and for disorders of the mouth and throat. Leclerc considered hypericum to be analgesic, anti-inflammatory and noted that its antibiotic activity was concentrated in the fruits. Other French phytotherapists have combined hypericum oil with camphor essential oil, as a rub in painful rheumatic conditions. Internal uses in France have included asthma, bronchitis, chronic cystitis, digestive disorders and worms.

In Portugal, reflecting mainly French and Spanish practice, the herb has been thought to stimulate appetite and promote digestion, to relieve coughs and topically to heal and cicatrise or tighten up wounds.[10] In Spain, the leading Spanish phytotherapist P. Font Quer[11] noted that so many virtues had been attributed to the plant that it was prudent to list none but its key uses as a wound and burn healer, and as a remedy for bedwetting in children. Italian usage closely resembles that of other Latin countries, though the herb has also been used to lower high blood pressure.[12] It has been and still is extensively used in Russia, for problems including bronchial asthma, peptic ulcer, diseases of the liver and bile ducts, rheumatic aches and pains and shingles.

Around the world—a brief review

Hypericum flourishes in many areas of the world and its virtues as a medicine have been utilised in north Africa, South Africa, the Middle East, northern India, Australia and New Zealand, as well as the Americas and Europe. Several of the 370 species of hypericum are also used medicinally, and some are being actively researched, especially those that have figured in traditional Chinese medicine and in *kampo*, Japanese traditional medicine.

In north Africa, hypericum is native to the higher regions of Tunisia and Morocco, where it has been primarily used to heal wounds and burns, and for digestive disorders.[13] In southern Anatolia in Turkey, it has been taken as a decoction or infusion for stomach ache.[14] Several other species of hypericum found in Turkey are also used medicinally. Within Ayurvedic medicine, the main traditional medicine of India, *Hypericum perforatum* has much the same actions as those found in Europe: astringent, anthelmintic (worming agent), emmenagogue, diuretic and wound healer.[15]

IMPORTANT COMBINATIONS WITH OTHER HERBAL MEDICINES

The art of the herbalist lies largely in selecting appropriate herbs to complement, modify or mitigate the effects of the leading herb(s) chosen for the prescription, which of course must meet the needs identified for the patient concerned. As a result hypericum can figure in a bewilderingly large number of therapeutic situations, depending on its role within the prescription. That being said, hypericum combines particularly well with the four herbs described here. Each one of them complements a different aspect of hypericum's repertoire as a medicine. Three of the four are well researched herbs, and their therapeutic activity is clearly understood. Black cohosh is not so well researched, though there is significant evidence to support its use during the menopause.

Black cohosh (*Cimicifuga racemosa*)
With oestrogenic, anti-inflammatory and nervine properties, black cohosh makes an ideal partner with hypericum for menopausal problems such as nervous exhaustion, depression, and hot flushing. Hypericum may possibly have an hormonal effect, but it certainly does not compare with the significant oestrogenic activity conferred on *Cimicifuga* by its steroidal saponins, constituents which have a structure very similar to the body's own steroid hormones. A native North American plant, black cohosh seems able to help the body adjust to the hormonal changes that occur at menopause, in particular the fall-off in oestrogen levels. In one clinical study the combination of hypericum and black cohosh was shown to bring relief in most cases of hot flushing (78 per cent), and of reduced concentration (61 per cent) in 812 menopausal women.[16] In another study 81 per cent rated the combination as 'good to very good' for problems linked to the menopause.[17] The combination is useful, too, for rheumatic and arthritic problems, whether occurring around the menopause or not, both herbs reducing inflammation and easing stiffness and pain; and it can be valuable for anxiety, panic and headaches, as black cohosh is markedly sedative. The normal weekly dose of each herb in combination is about 20–25g of hypericum and 5–15g of black cohosh—taken as extracts, capsules or tinctures.

Echinacea (*Echinacea* spp.—*angustifolia*, *purpurea* and *pallida*)
The foremost herb for raising the body's immune resistance, echinacea is commonly used to treat viral and bacterial infections such as colds, flus and tonsillitis, and chronic problems such as acne, thrush, and chronic fatigue syndrome. Though it has not been as

well researched as hypericum, there is clear-cut evidence that it stimulates resistance to infection, in particular upper respiratory problems such as influenza.[18] Significantly, it also has anti-inflammatory and wound-healing properties.

Working principally as an immune stimulant, and aiding in infection through improved white blood cell function, it complements hypericum's antiviral and anti-depressant activity very well. In fact, echinacea, like hypericum, can be thought of as an 'anti-immune depressant'. Together they make a good combination for herpes sores and other herpetic infection such as shingles. For hepatitis B or C this combination is a good starting-point before being able to get professional herbal or naturopathic advice. In HIV infection there is some controversy over the value of echinacea, so always consult a herbal or naturopathic practitioner. This combination is likely to prove effective for people who are run down and 'under the weather', constantly getting one cold after another. Stress and stressful events have recently been shown to be a major factor in depressing immune resistance to the point where a cold sets in. Hypericum, with its nerve tonic activity, can be very helpful in this context. Chronic infection, and the experience of being ill over a long period of time, both often produce a depressed mental state—again indicating hypericum. It is probably easiest to take hypericum and echinacea as extracts in tablet form, though they can just as easily be taken as capsules and tinctures. Weekly doses would normally be 20–25g of hypericum and 10–15g of echinacea.

Gingko (*Ginkgo biloba*)

Ginkgo was Germany's top-selling medicine in 1993 and is taken by huge numbers of people from the age of 50 onwards to maintain the circulation to the brain and to protect against dementia and nerve damage. A 1997 article in the *Journal of the American Medical Association*, reporting a 52-week long clinical trial, concluded that gingko appeared to stabilise demented states, and in a significant number of patients to improve both mental and social function.[19] The oldest surviving species of tree on the planet, and native to China, ginkgo has been intensively researched and has a staggeringly large number of potential uses as a medicine: for poor memory, depression, sudden deafness, tinnitus, multiple sclerosis, pre-menstrual problems, erectile dysfunction and eczema, to name only a few. Given its remarkable ability to support blood flow through the cerebral circulation, its anti-inflammatory and protective roles on nerve and other tissue, and its pronounced anti-dementia activity, ginkgo is perhaps a specific remedy for older people. As depression and many nervous disorders occur more frequently in older people, a combination of ginkgo and hypericum offers distinct advantages over hypericum alone. Both are readily available in tablet form (I would usually recommend standardised extracts for self-medication) and can be safely taken together long term.

Valerian (*Valeriana officinalis*)

A native European plant, valerian has been much investigated and figures in many of the world's pharmacopoeias. Its longstanding use in herbal medicine as a relaxing sedative—for nervous overactivity, anxiety and related problems such as insomnia and tight-chestedness—has been confirmed. It has been shown to promote sleep, to improve sleep quality, and to have no negative impact on people's use of machinery (for example, driving), as alcohol does. A number of clinical trials have used a combined hypericum and valerian extract to treat anxiety states, with notable success. In one reported in the section on Anxiety (see p. 51),[20] the combined extract proved more effective than diazepam after two weeks of treatment. This combination used a very low dose of hypericum, which suggests that hypericum and valerian may enhance each other's effect. In a more recent trial the combined extract proved to be as effective as amitryptiline.[21]

Certainly, whenever anxiety and depression are present together, these two herbs are strongly indicated, helping to improve mood, slow down nervous overactivity and encourage a more refreshing sleep. Hypericum can be taken at a standard dosage, with a valerian preparation—tablet, capsule, tincture or infusion—taken at the same time or just at night as required. A slight word of *caution*: valerian is an extremely safe herb, but different people have different sensitivities to it. When taking it for the first time, start with the lowest dose. If you experience no initial effect increase the dose until its gentle sedative activity becomes apparent (up to the maximum recommended dosage).

*   *   *

Although these combinations can be used to self-medicate, it is often better to get the advice of an experienced medical herbalist. In complex or chronic cases the combination of several herbs is often preferable to one or two alone, each herb being chosen for its specific therapeutic effect (for example, sedative) as well as for its ability to complement the activity of the other herbs within the prescription. Note that some of these herbal medicines *will* interact with orthodox medicines—for example, ginkgo will increase the action of anti-coagulants such as Warfarin. *If you are self-medicating, be sure to consult your doctor or herbalist and follow the recommendations on the label.*

CHAPTER 8

Hypericum as a Medicine

The air was heavy with the smell of resin and a gentle breeze from the fields rocked the horsetails. With her swarthy hands Grandmother started picking herbs, and at the same time she told me all about the healing properties of St John's wort.

Maxim Gorky, My Apprenticeship

Putting the pieces of the jigsaw back together, and trying to create a balanced view of hypericum and its range of medicinal uses, is not that straightforward. The wealth of data is now so large that it is hard to step back and get a clear view of the plant as a whole. Each year journal articles identify new potential applications for hypericum's anti-depressant or antiviral activity, and new active constituents with novel potential uses are discovered. The variety and rate of growth of information is astonishing, sometimes bewildering, and it is hard to know how much weight to give to different pieces of research, especially as they are sometimes contradictory. In this situation, one can take the plunge and attempt to paint a coherent picture of the herb *as a whole*—perhaps inevitably making mistakes along the way—or one must accept that such a project is hopeless, and that knowledge is made up of lots of disconnected slivers of information.

HYPERICUM AS A MEDICINE—AN OVERVIEW

Twenty-five years ago you would only have found hypericum being used to treat depression in the surgeries of phytotherapists or herbalists. Today, hypericum's value as an *anti-depressant* is beyond dispute: mild to moderate depression, low self-esteem, fear and nervous exhaustion lie at the heart of the herb's efficacy as a medicine. With diverse, subtle effects on the central nervous system, and on serotonin levels especially, it may also be of value in problems as varied as eating disorders, addictions, insomnia, headaches, and hyperactivity in children. On its own, and especially in combination with valerian, it works as an *anxiolytic*, relieving anxiety, panic and related problems. In combination with black cohosh it appears to bring consistent relief to menopausal symptoms such as hot flushes and tiredness, and it may possibly help in pre-menstrual syndrome where depression is a regular feature.

At the same time it has significant *antimicrobial* and *antiviral* properties and exerts what can best be described as a tonic or stimulant activity on the immune system: it finds use in infection caused by enveloped viruses (some herpes viruses being present in the majority of the population), including HIV, HCV, shingles and flu. Its effect on the immune system, and its photochemical activity, mean that the herb (more specifically, hypericin) may have a role as a precisely targeted antiviral and *anti-cancer agent*, switched on by photoluminescence once within affected tissue. The herb as a whole has significant *antioxidant* activity, and combined with antiviral and anti-cancer effects, could have value as a prophylactic or preventative against cancer. It may prove beneficial in chronic disease of all kinds.

Due especially to its high content of proanthocyanidins, it acts as a *cardiotonic* and *vasodilator*, supporting the heart and circulation and conferring these protective effects on conditions such as angina, chronic heart failure and arteriosclerosis. With both local and systemic *anti-inflammatory* activity, hypericum may be of value in chronic inflammatory conditions, particularly autoimmune conditions such as Crohn's disease and rheumatoid arthritis. There are indications that the herb has a *liver protective* role. It stimulates bile production (choleretic), supporting liver detoxification and improving fat absorption.

Extracts of the herb taken internally, and the oil applied topically, aid *wound and tissue repair*, in particular on the skin and within the gut. They are *astringent* and have *analgesic* activity, making them useful in stomach ulcers and haemorrhoids, neuralgic problems such as sciatica, to speed recovery from operations and dental extractions, and for wounds, minor burns and the like.

Finally, hypericum can be used to enhance health and performance, rather than to treat illness. It appears to improve stamina in athletes and in several clinical trials improved cognitive function in depressed patients (see chapter 9).

All in all, a formidable picture for a humble wort! Hypericum is a natural anti-depressant, and it is also *much more*—a healer of wounds, both physical and emotional, with *protective* or *preventative* activity against a variety of disorders. However, hypericum is not, as Paracelsus claimed, a universal panacea. It has, or may be proven to have, medicinal value in the conditions listed above, but in several cases this reflects the inadequacy of existing treatments rather than a powerful therapeutic action on the part of hypericum.

Key uses

- Mild to moderate depression, despondency, SAD, anxiety, panic, fear; related problems such as nervous exhaustion, insomnia, headaches; improves motivation, concentration and emotional stability.
- Viral infection: HIV and AIDS, hepatitis C, glandular fever, influenza, herpes simplex sores, shingles.
- Repair of wounds and damaged tissue; gastritis and dyspepsia, stomach ulcers; irritable and inflammatory bowel disorders.
- Topically (mainly the oil): bruises, cuts, abrasions, small wounds, bites, whitlows, operation scars, burns, tooth extractions, leg ulcers, haemorrhoids. Also neuralgic problems: sciatica, shingles, toothache, trigeminal neuralgia.

Other uses (*less well investigated, or less significant, uses*)

- Addictions, attention deficit disorder, 'burn-out', eating disorders, other stress disorders; chronic pain.
- Menopausal problems, especially exhaustion; pre-menstrual syndrome.
- Liver protective activity; disorders of liver and gall bladder.
- Cardiotonic and vasodilator—support for heart and circulation when under stress.
- Urinary disorders, especially urinary incontinence; in children, bedwetting.
- Inflammatory conditions, e.g. rheumatoid arthritis; other auto-immune disease.
- Possible cancer treatment; cancer prevention.
- Chronic ill health in general.

DOSAGE AND PREPARATIONS

The right dose for hypericum depends entirely on the preparation used—infusion, tincture, standardised extract, or oil. In most cases the standard dose is appropriate for all conditions.

*   *   *

Parts used: fresh or dried flowering tops of the plant, with buds, flowers and seed capsules present.

Standard recommended doses

Infusion	2–4g of dried herb.[1] Use 1 teaspoonful per cup (about 200ml of water); infuse herb for 10 minutes in a closed container. Take 2–3 cups a day. If using fresh herb, use double the quantity. The optimum temperature for infusions is 80°C (175°F).[2]

Powder	2–4g a day. Take in capsules or with water in 2–3 divided doses.
Tincture (1:5)	2–4ml three times a day with water.[3] Take diluted with water.
	Can be simply prepared: put 50g of fresh flowering tops and 250ml of vodka or brandy (i.e. 40 per cent alcohol) together in an airtight container. Shake and leave for ten days, shaking once each day. Strain, pour into dark glass bottles, and label.
Fluid extract (1:1)	0.5–1ml[3] (approx. 10 to 20 drops) three times a day. Take diluted with water.
Standardised extract	Equivalent to 0.5–3.0mg total hypericin a day.[3] Take as recommended on packaging. For 300mg tablets or capsules take three times a day.
Oil	1 teaspoonful on an empty stomach, morning and evening.[4] (See below for preparation.)

External applications
(normally applied 2–3 times a day)

Oil	Rub gently into affected area; for greater effect warm area with hot water bottle first, e.g. in muscular pains or sciatica.
Compress	Apply firmly on to affected area. Use sterilised gauze or other lint-free cloth soaked in hot/warm infusion.
Gargle/mouthwash	Use 50–100ml of infusion (hot or cold) and rinse round mouth or gargle. May be swallowed.

General advice on dosage

The above dosages are appropriate for adults who are self-medicating for any reason—mild to moderate depression, SAD, menopausal problems and so on. Hypericum is very safe, so if after about six weeks the standard dose does not seem to work, you can try taking more—up to about a third more. Similarly, if you need less than the standard dose to achieve the desired effect, reduce the dosage: in some clinical trials patients successfully reduced the dosage after three to four weeks. Higher doses do not necessarily mean greater effectiveness, and *in illness such as severe depression, HIV/AIDS and hepatitis C, where a higher dose is required, hypericum should only be taken on the advice of a health care professional.*

People aged 65 and over may need less than the standard adult dose and are recommended to start treatment with about two-thirds of the dose, increasing to the standard dose if necessary.

Children can be given hypericum, typically for bedwetting, as a mild sedative, and to reduce restlessness.[5] Young children can be given about one cup of infusion or ten drops of fluid extract a day;[5] children aged between 6 and 12 years should be given half the adult dose.[1] *In most cases, especially if the condition is more than short-term, Hypericum should be taken only on the advice of an appropriate health care practitioner. Some authorities recommend its use in children only under medical supervision.*[1]

If you are already taking medicines, especially anti-depressants, please read the section on Interactions (p. 111).

Preparation of hypericum oil

Making hypericum oil could not be simpler, and will provide you with an effective household remedy for cuts, wounds, burns, toothache and the like. Many different processes are recommended for making the oil, each producing slightly different results.

Contrary to received opinion, the oil does not contain hypericin, though it does contain hypericin-breakdown products which are partly responsible for its colour. The oil also contains hyperforin, flavonoids and xanthones. If you want to use the oil for wound-healing, it is best to expose the herb to sunlight as 'the presence of light during preparation of the oil increases its flavonoid concentration'[6]—a further link between hypericum and the sun.

*   *   *

Method 1. This traditional method is very straightforward. On a dry, sunny morning pick about 100g (4oz) of fresh buds, flowers and seed capsules of St John's wort. Chop up and place in a clear glass jar that can be sealed—a Kilner jar or similar. Cover the herb with 1 litre (1¾ pints) of virgin olive oil, seal tightly and shake well to remove air pockets. Ensure that the herb is entirely covered with oil (if not, it will produce mould growth and ruin the oil), and leave to macerate in a sunny site for three to four weeks, e.g. on a window-sill. In a matter of days the dark green olive oil should start to turn deep crimson red as the hypericin-breakdown products begin to dissolve into the oil. The darker red the colour, the better the oil is thought to be. Strain the oil and pour into small sterilised dark glass bottles. Labels the bottles clearly. Store in a cool, dark place. If wanted, the strained oil can be used with a fresh supply of St John's wort, going through the whole process again to produce a stronger oil.

*   *   *

Method 2. As before take 100g (4oz) of buds, flowers and seed capsules. Chop up and place in a sealable clear glass jar. Cover the herb with 500 ml (1 pint) of virgin olive oil and 500ml (1 pint) of white wine. Leave to macerate in sunlight for three days. Put in a double boiler (bain-marie) and gently evaporate the wine. Strain and bottle up as for Method 1. This makes a double-strength oil in one go, ready for use within three days. This method was developed earlier this century by the French phytotherapist Leclerc, after more than ten years researching hypericum's role as a wound and burn treatment.

*   *   *

These oils can be kept for use for up to 12 months provided they are properly stored. For minor burns, the simple and thorough recommendations given by the German phytotherapist, Dr P. Schilcher, should be followed:

> The scalded or burned areas should be cooled immediately at the accident site by immersing in cold water or pouring this over for several minutes. Local treatment with hypericum oil may then follow. Place sterile gauze soaked in the 'red oil' on the burned areas. Renew the oil dressing after about 10 hours.[5]

Hypericum oil can be used as a base for mixing with essential oils such as camphor. I have found the following to be particularly effective for arthritic and rheumatic pains:

Hypericum oil   100ml

Add essential oils of:

Ginger   1ml (or 20 drops)
Juniper   1ml
Lavender   1ml
Wintergreen   1ml

Shake bottle thoroughly and label it. Rub firmly into stiff and painful areas. For best results apply after a bath, or warm affected area with a hot water bottle first.

Quality is everything—buying hypericum over the counter

Everybody familiar with the world of herbal medicine knows that the effectiveness of a herb depends entirely on its quality—the care that has been put in to growing, harvesting and processing it. Poor-quality material at whatever the price is a waste of money. There is no point in buying suspiciously cheap mail-order supplies of hypericum, for you are likely to be throwing your money away; and worse, by taking poor-quality herbal medicine you are less likely to get better, delaying effective treatment and probably leading you to doubt the herb's therapeutic value.

A consumer survey released by the US Good Housekeeping Institute in March 1998, revealed some shocking statistics that confirm the importance of using good-quality plant material. The Good Housekeeping team analysed the composition of a range of hypericum products available over the counter in the US.[7] They discovered:

- A *17-fold* difference between capsules containing the smallest amount of hypericin and those containing the largest amount, based on manufacturer's recommended dosage.
- A *13-fold* difference in pseudohypericin in the capsules.
- A *7–8 fold* differential from the highest to the lowest levels of liquid extracts.

Although some of this extreme variation between products would be due to the natural variability of plant material, buying hypericum over the counter is not far short of a consumer's nightmare: those products at the lower end of the scale may well have been worthless as medicines. Quality-control procedures for herbal medicines in Europe, Australia and New Zealand are generally better than in the USA—hypericum is sold in these countries mostly as a medicine rather than a food supplement—but there is *no* automatic guarantee that what you buy will contain good-quality plant material.

Following a few simple rules should, however, mean that you purchase hypericum of an appropriate quality—to suit your needs and your pocket.

- The simplest but most expensive way to take hypericum is as a standardised extract, which generally guarantees quality with a minimum level of hypericin. So far no standardised extracts are available which have been organically grown. A number of good-quality products (all tablets) are available, including Kira (Lichtwer

Pharma), Quest, and Holland & Barrett's own brand.

- Buying certified organically-grown hypericum offers a different type of quality from that of a standardised extract. Always try to buy organically grown herb. Reject material that is faded or discoloured, or contains leaf and stem, with few petals or seed capsules. Buy from reputable suppliers.
- Tinctures and fluid extracts are versatile preparations, useful for combining with other herbs. They contain alcohol. Buy from reputable suppliers or a well-known brand.
- *Avoid* herbal medicines sold by mail order unless you know the company supplies good-quality preparations. Many contain poor-quality powder or extract, or have far too little herb to produce the desired effect.
- Look for a crimson red colour when buying hypericum oil.
- Growing and harvesting your own plants is the cheapest way to take hypericum, but make sure you start with authenticated plants or seeds. Some varieties of *hypericum perforatum* have a low level of active constituents; preferably one should grow the southern European narrow-leaved variety *var. angustifolia*. Harvest, dry and store with care.

Store all hypericum products in a cool place and out of direct sunlight.

SAFETY ISSUES

Hypericum's safety record is one vital reason for its popularity as an anti-depressant. That said, as with any medication, it does produce unwanted effects in some people, and does not suit everyone who takes it. Moreover, there are situations where taking hypericum might be inadvisable, as very little is yet known about the herb's potential to interact with other medicines.

Side-effects

'Side-effects are rare and mild', noted the authors of the 1996 study of hypericum in the *British Medical Journal*.[8] This is a fair summary, reflecting the fact that more than 20 million people in Germany have now taken hypericum extracts for 12 months or more; but it does not mean that hypericum is altogether free from side-effects. The commonest reported side-effects, taken from a clinical study[9] involving 3,250 patients, are:

- gastrointestinal symptoms (0.55%)—nausea [6], abdominal pains [5], loss of appetite [3], diarrhoea [2], unspecified [2];
- allergic reactions (0.52%)—allergy [6], skin rash [6], itchiness [5];
- fatigue (0.40%);
- anxiety (0.26%);
- dizziness (0.15%);
- other side-effects (0.55%).

(Figures in brackets = number of cases (total = 79))

Additionally, 1.5 per cent (48) of patients discontinued treatment reporting a roughly similar picture of side-effects.

Side-effects seem to occur more frequently early on in treatment, often stopping as hypericum's anti-depressant activity starts to work—usually after two to three weeks. If you find that you are getting mild side-effects, then it is worth continuing and seeing whether they slowly wear off. If they are causing you a problem, stop taking the herb and see your herbal or medical practitioner.

In contrast to the above statistics, the 1996 *BMJ* study, reviewing 23 clinical trials, found side-effects occurring in 19.8 per cent of those taking hypericum and 35.9 per cent of those taking synthetic anti-depressants! To some this may simply confirm the old adage of 'lies, damn lies and statistics', but in fact this shows that people report side-effects for different reasons, and that the number of side-effects does not tell you about differences in their severity. In some clinical trials patients will be strongly urged to report even trivial symptoms, in others they may be discouraged from reporting severe side-effects due to embarrassment or lack of confidence in the practitioner.

Gaining a precise picture of the frequency of side-effects associated with hypericum is therefore difficult. Nevertheless, one can say with certainty that hypericum has dramatically fewer side-effects than synthetic anti-depressants, and rarely produces anything other than mild disturbance. As mentioned at the beginning of the book, hypericum caused fewer 'side-effects' than placebos, in 15 clinical trials.[10] Research looking at hypericum's potential to cause cellular damage leading to cancer is also very reassuring. The following quote may not be grammatical, but it gets the message over! There is 'completely no indication of a mutagenic potential of hypericum extract'.[11]

Finally, and perhaps most important of all, when side-effects do occur they are reversible, fading away once hypericum treatment is stopped.[12]

Contraindications

None are known,[1] though fair-skinned people should be careful about sunbathing and ultraviolet light treatment, when taking hypericum.

Some fair-skinned individuals taking a high dose standardised extract (600mg of hypericum three times a day) suffered from mild redness to the skin after 15 days' treatment, and showed a significant reduction (28 per cent) in the amount of UV light (UVA) needed to stimulate pigmentation.[13] This is not a recommendation to use hypericum as a suntanning aid!

Interactions/Changing anti-depressants

None have been reported.[1] Despite hypericum's safety as a medicine, however, one should nevertheless be cautious about taking it with other anti-depressants. Interaction between hypericum and synthetic anti-depressants is theoretically possible but unproven. Until further research is done, no one knows for certain what risks are involved. You are therefore recommended to follow some simple advice:

- If already taking an anti-depressant, do *not* suddenly stop taking it.
- Do not take hypericum with MAO inhibitors such as Nardil (phenelzine) or Parnate (tranylcypromine). MAOIs can evoke serious side-effects, and might interact with hypericum. Taking the two together is not worth the risk.
- If taking an SSRI anti-depressant it is *probably* all right to phase this out while simultaneously building up to the standard dosage of hypericum. *Discuss this with your health care provider first*, and be careful not to overdose.

Though unlikely, hypericum may interact with other prescription drugs. It is sensible to inform your doctor or health care professional when starting treatment with hypericum.

Hypericum during pregnancy and lactation
Taking any medication during pregnancy and while breastfeeding is to be avoided unless clearly necessary, and hypericum is no exception. Take only on the advice of a medical or herbal practitioner.

Over and above this, however, there are concerns that hypericum might stimulate uterine muscle contraction and increase risks of miscarriage. Such fears are, I believe, mistaken and based on a misunderstanding of hypericum's effect on uterine muscle tone.

Concerns were first raised after publication of research in 1981, which investigated the 'uterotonic' action of infusions of nine different medicinal plants.[14] Two of these—linseed (*Linum usitatissimum*) and bearberry (*Arctostaphylos uva-ursi*)—produced no increase in muscle tone at all. Of the remaining seven herbs, hypericum had the least effect of all on uterine muscle tone. The herb with the greatest stimulant activity proved to be chamomile (*Chamomilla recutita*), which is commonly drunk as an infusion during pregnancy to relieve nausea and morning sickness. Chamomile has an almost complete absence of side-effects, and the *British Herbal Compendium*[15] lists just 'extremely rare contact allergy' under side-effects for the herb. Furthermore, the research tested the plants' activity *in vitro*, and it is always difficult to generalise from labora-tory-based experiments to clinical reality. Put in this context, it is clear that hypericum is very safe, although it should still be used with caution if trying to conceive, during pregnancy (especially during the first three months), and if breastfeeding.

Another way to look at the issue, of course, is to compare the reported side-effects of hypericum with other equivalent treatment. If you have to take an anti-depressant or an antiviral then, in most cases, hypericum will prove by far the safest option.

Consulting a professional herbal practitioner

Self-treatment is fine provided one does not start to get truly ill, for it then becomes harder and harder to make the right decisions about what to do next. This is particularly so for depression, as morale, will and self-confidence seep away. Taking hypericum is an excellent start for treating depression and other disorders, but if it does not prove sufficient on its own, consulting a professional herbal practitioner (or phytotherapist) is a sensible next step, giving you sound advice on natural treatments for your condition—diet, supplements, herbal medicines, relaxation and exercise.

Some medical practitioners have trained in herbal medicine, but in most countries they are a very small minority and hard to find. To get advice about herbal medicine, you are usually best off seeing a medical herbalist who will as a minimum have completed four years of training in herbal medicine, often at BSc (Hons) level. He or she will have a good understanding of physiology and pathology, and be able to make a diagnosis. If the practitioner is worried that you might have a serious health problem, you will be referred for further investigations or to your doctor, but usually treatment is provided on the spot.

As I hope has become clear in this book, herbal medicines are very different from synthetic, chemical medicines. Though few herbs have been as intensively researched as hypericum, most herbal medicines are extremely safe and rarely produce side-effects. One reason for this is that they work with the body's own self-correcting processes rather than overriding them. By

113

combining several different herbs the practitioner is able to select herbs that work together in a variety of related ways—for example, to relieve skin irritation, reduce inflammation, detoxify and ease anxiety in conditions such as eczema. The overall effect produced then supports the body's own attempts to recover good health. For more information on how to find a medical herbalist, please see Useful Addresses.

CHAPTER 9

The Future

Slowly, and thanks in large part to hypericum, the Western world is beginning to wake up to the therapeutic potential of plant medicines. There is absolutely no doubt that they will have a crucial role to play in the medicine of the twenty-first century. Used appropriately, they are:

Gentle-acting and effective
While mainstream medicine is excellent at responding to medical emergencies, saving lives and dealing with acute illness, it is far less effective, and at times potentially dangerous, when it comes to treating chronic ill health. As people live longer and the elderly make up a greater and greater proportion of the population of Western societies, chronic illnesses, especially degenerative disorders, will become more prevalent. Such health problems require gentle-acting and safe treatment, similar to hypericum's profile in treating depression.

It is a fairly well-kept secret in most English-speaking countries that in much of Europe, and particularly in Germany, gentle-acting and effective herbal extracts are already the standard first-choice treatment for chronic conditions as diverse as varicose veins, angina and mild chronic heart failure, early senile dementia, memory loss, insomnia, anxiety and stress, dyspepsia and flatulence, and enlarged prostate. All these conditions have been shown to respond well to herbal medicines with a minimum of side-effects.

Why the German-speaking medical world should utilise these botanical drugs, while the English-speaking world is hooked almost exclusively to synthetic drugs, remains something of a mystery. One can deduce that culture, and political and financial interests, have at least as much to do with developments in medicine as clinical and laboratory research!

Cost-effective

Research having confirmed hypericum's value as an anti-depressant, health care purchasers and providers are now beginning to do some simple arithmetic.

In the UK, the number of prescriptions written for synthetic anti-depressants *doubled* between 1991 and 1997 from around 8.5 million to over 16 million. About four million people in the UK now take anti-depressants each year. The overall cost to the National Health Service (NHS) was £239 million in 1997, up from £54 million in 1991. The fourfold increase in cost reflects not just the doubling in number of prescriptions but the increased use and greater cost of SSRIs such as Prozac. While a month's supply of Prozac costs the NHS £20.77, older 'tricyclic' anti-depressants are far cheaper—Prothiaden costs £4.20 per month. In comparison, the monthly cost of standardised extracts of hypericum, at the prices that the NHS would be able to agree, is probably less than £4.20[1]—the current wholesale price of the herb is after all £5.50 per kilo.

In the USA there is already talk of the cost savings that can accrue from using hypericum and other medicinal plants. An article in *Medical Sciences Bulletin* in March 1998 notes that 'studies have been published in respected journals demonstrating that herbal remedies are both safe and effective'. It then details St John's wort's effectiveness as a medicine and states:

Equally important in this era of managed care is the cost savings associated with Hypericum when compared with the commonly prescribed anti-depressant Prozac. A one month's supply of Prozac costs $72, whereas Hypericum costs less than $9 a month. If Hypericum were shown to be effective in 25% of depressed patients, a health maintenance organisation spending $1,000,000 a year on anti-depressants could recognise a saving of $250,000 per year.[2]

If this were not a powerful enough argument on its own, the article goes on to calculate the cost savings that could be made by utilising other herbal medicines such as ginger (*Zingiber officinale*) as an anti-emetic, nettle (*Urtica dioica*) for its anti-allergy activity and peppermint oil (*Mentha piperita*) for irritable bowel syndrome. It estimates that savings on the annual drugs bill would be between $500,000 and $750,000. For health care managers this is powerful stuff, especially when you add in the fact that hypericum causes few side-effects. If the current multi-centre comparative study of hypericum, coordinated by the Duke University Medical Center in North Carolina, produces positive results, hypericum will in no time be widely prescribed as an anti-depressant in the USA.

With a 'foot in the door', there will quickly be a well-worn track across the threshold as other well-researched herbal medicines make a rather sudden transition from being quaint or obsolete folk remedies to 'state of the art' medicines. This is not a rash prediction—several major US pharmaceutical companies are already gearing up to produce prescription herbal medicines.

Increased patient choice

Hypericum's proven safety record makes it very suitable for self-treatment and in the process can give significant control and self-responsibility back to the patient. With few problems associated with its use, hypericum can be safely self-medicated for mild depressive illness, SAD, anxiety, insomnia, and so on, allowing people to maintain their normal lives and independence.

Patient autonomy is clearly one reason why herbal medicines have become so popular; though the fact that over the last 50 years the medical profession has focused on technical developments in medicine at the expense of the therapeutic relationship is another factor. People with moderate to severe depression must of course see a health care practitioner, but most depressive illness is, fortunately, at the mild end of the spectrum.

Ecologically and environmentally safe

A further way in which medicine in the twenty-first century will steadily grow to rely on herbal medicines results from their having no harmful environmental impact. They cause no ecological damage if properly cultivated and no novel potentially dangerous compounds are released in their production. While herbs such as hypericum are totally integrated into the external environment, they are by and large equally well adapted to the *internal* environment of the body, especially the gastro-intestinal tract which, though we may not recognise it, is really a part of the 'outside' world rather than a part of our 'insides'!

Unlike drugs such as aspirin and antibiotics which can cause major problems within the gastro-intestinal tract, for example by killing off the bacteria or gut flora in our intestines, herbal medicines appear to actively support a healthy gut flora and gut membrane. In hypericum's case many of its actions—astringent, antimicrobial, tissue-healing, anti-inflammatory and antioxidant—will specifically promote the healthy self-repair of the gut wall membrane, which is normally replaced every four days.

Source of new medicines

As understanding of human physiology and of its extreme complexity grows, one hopes researchers will recognise that the 'magic bullet' approach to treatment is often unsuitable, sometimes causing as much or more of a problem than the illness being treated. Powerful, potentially toxic drugs—synthetic or herbal—may well be necessary in life-threatening or severe acute illness but in other less pressing situations more subtle approaches to treatment are indicated.

The great strength of herbal medicines is that, like the human body, they too are extremely complex natural substances, often able to influence body function without disrupting it. The many different small-scale influences exerted on the body by hypericum add up in total to a remarkable therapeutic effect. It is thought that many herbs work by this summation of subtle physiological effects. Ignoring such subtle effects means not seeing the thera-peutic richness that plant medicines offer.

Whether this view, common to those familiar with herbal medi-cines, will become more readily acknowledged is open to question. Current views on the role of 'natural products' see them as largely the repository of new, isolated 'magic bullets', isolated plant con-stituents that can be synthesised. Here is a good summary of this perspective:

> Until the middle of this century, development of medical treatment for human disease was intimately connected with the plant kingdom. Despite advances of the last three decades in utilising chemical synthetic approaches to drug design and sophisticated structure-activity studies, there is still a great need for novel compounds with unique mechanisms of action in the field of medicine . . . Major breakthroughs have resulted primarily from the study of natural products. Some of our most valuable drugs have been isolated from plant and animal sources, including aspirin, morphine, reserpine (the first anti-psychotic), almost all of our antibiotics, digitalis, and such anti-cancer agents as vincristine, vinblastine, and taxol. Recent political and social events suggest that new emphasis will be placed on natural products research in the years to come.[3]

NEW USES

Antiviral uses

Ongoing research continues to explore the use of hypericum and more particularly hypericin in viral infection, and as a potential anti-cancer treatment. As we saw in chapters 4 and 5, hypericin has an astonishing range of actions, and it would be surprising if evidence for use of hypericum, and its constituent, in severe ill-nesses such as HIV and hepatitis did not grow rapidly. Combi-nations of the two are being tried in trials on HIV and hepatitis

C, and hypericin's photoluminescent activity ensures that it will continue to receive much attention.

One of the least expected conditions which might benefit is multiple sclerosis (MS). Results of a study conducted by the US National Institute of Neurological Disorders and Stroke provides new evidence of the role of viral triggers in MS, and may eventually lead to clinical trials using antiherpetic agents as a treatment. In the study, over 70 per cent of patients with the relapsing-remitting form of MS showed an increased immune response to human herpes virus-6 (HHV-6), while approximately 35 per cent of MS patients studied had detectable levels of active HHV-6 in their serum. Scientists believe that there may be a point in time during the development of MS when the virus, which lies dormant in the body for years, reactivates, accounting for its presence in a subset of MS patients. If this is the case then, given the antiherpetic activity of hypericum and hypericin, they could become useful medicines in certain cases of MS.[4]

Pain relief and poor impulse control
Despite the fact that hypericum's ability to relieve pain lies at the core of its use in herbal medicine and homoeopathy, this aspect of the herb has been poorly investigated—neuralgia including sciatica, painful inflammatory states, and chronic pain of any kind being typical applications. As with its anti-depressant activity, hypericum is likely to work in several different ways to relieve pain. It may, for example, have a direct action on opioid receptors,[5] though another mechanism to be considered is related to the link between good-quality sleep, especially stage IV deep sleep, and serotonin and endorphin levels. Raised serotonin levels increase time spent in deep sleep, leading to increased endorphin production and muscle relaxation.[6] Endorphins are the body's natural painkillers with profound analgesic and relaxant activity affecting the body and mind as a whole. Lowered levels lead to increased pain sensation. When one considers that SSRI anti-depressants have been successfully used to treat chronic pain, chronic headaches,

phantom limb pain and diabetic neuropathy,[6] the empirical use of hypericum to relieve pain seems spot-on.

Significantly, alcohol, benzodiazepine drugs and possibly narcotic pain-killers all lower endorphin levels.[6] This suggests a possible way in which hypericum could aid withdrawal from addictions, helping here perhaps as much with emotional as with physical symptoms.

SSRIs have also been shown to have clinical value in what is known as 'poor impulse control', and have been used in anorexia nervosa, bulimia, obsessive-compulsive disorder and violent behaviour including suicide.[7] Speculative links have also been made between serotonin levels and schizophrenia. Given the herb's anti-depressant action, eating disorders might respond favourably to treatment with hypericum. Additionally, research into a Spanish species of hypericum (*H. caprifolium*) demonstrated that the plant had an anorexic action in animals.[8] Whether any of the other disorders listed might benefit is, at this moment, impossible to say.

Performance enhancer
Whether hypericum improves mental and physical performance in healthy people is likely to be a question raised repeatedly in coming years. Like herbs such as ginseng (*Panax ginseng*) and withania (*Withania somnifera*), there are signs that hypericum improves 'cognitive function'—overall mental performance, as well as athletic performance. In a recent randomised, double blind, placebo-controlled study, on well trained long-distance runners and triathletes, those who were given a combination of 170mg of hypericum extract, vitamin E and the minerals magnesium, potassium and silica showed a significant increase in aerobic efficiency (a raised anaerobic threshold) and reduced levels of lactic acid production.[9] Quite how St John's wort might contribute to this overall effect is hard to say, though the herb's cardiovascular activity, leading to improved perfusion, might be significant despite the low dosage of hypericum extract. Further research into this performance-enhancing activity of hypericum is under way.

As regards mental performance, in one clinical trial the cognitive function of 50 depressed patients was found to have increased significantly.[10] In a further trial, comparing the 'tricyclic' imipramine with hypericum, the herbal extract also improved cognitive function, this time in 24 healthy volunteers.[11]

Circadian rhythms

The physical and mental functioning of the body is regulated by circadian rhythms, the body's internal clock, which determine the timing and duration of high and low levels of hormones, neurotransmitters, etc., over a 24-hour cycle. Hopefully, future research into hypericum will throw more light on the herb's effects on natural biorhythms.

Directly or indirectly, hypericum influences melatonin release, the neurotransmitter centrally involved in ordering the daily cycle of sleep and wakefulness, and crucial in the regulation and synchronisation of other neurotransmitters, especially serotonin (with which it has an inverse relationship).[6] Hypericum of course has already been shown to positively affect serotonin, noradrenaline and dopamine levels, and interacts on a number of levels with the hypothalamic-pituitary-adrenal axis, the pathway at the heart of our response to stress.

Taken together, these effects suggest that hypericum might prove useful in a host of health problems linked to disordered circadian rhythms, the most obvious being jet lag, shift working and pre-menstrual syndrome (PMS).

Other uses

And finally, the most unexpected development of all? Following the traditional, magical use of the plant as a talisman to ward off and protect against evil, hypericum is now being recommended for its protective powers against 'harassing entities' in the book *How to Defend Yourself Against Alien Abduction*. Hypericum, it seems, has made it into the X-files. Whether this is an indication of its value in disconcerting extra-terrestrials, or a sign that it may be of use in paranoia, only time will tell![12]

STANDARDISED EXTRACTS

Much of the research published in 1998 shows convincingly that hyperforin is the key component of the herb linked to its anti-depressant effects. The limited research into hyperforin-standardised extracts to date suggests that they have a greater anti-depressant effect than hypericin-standardised extracts. In a trial that compared the two extracts, patients given the hyperforin extract (300mg hypericum extract with 0.5 per cent hyperforin) 'showed the largest anti-depressant effect, and demonstrated the lowest incidence of adverse events.'[13] One would therefore expect that within a relatively short space of time hyperforin-based extracts will be launched onto the market, for although hypericum extracts have stronger anti-depressant activity than hyperforin on its own, this constituent is likely to be seen as the new 'marker' for the herb's use as an anti-depressant. The recommendation has already been made that extracts should be standardised at 3 per cent hyperforin.[14]

When available, hyperforin-standardised extracts will be preferable to hypericin-standardised extracts for depression and related disorders, though the hypericin extract will continue to be more useful where an antiviral activity is required. With a little luck, however, a more sophisticated approach will be employed.

> It is becoming clear, therefore, that standardising the therapeutically used extracts on one single class of constituents is not sufficient, and that efforts should be made to identify and evaluate the relative therapeutic importance of various extract components and to study possible pharmacological interactions.[15]

These researchers are clearly willing to grapple with the complexity of the herb, and should new standardised extracts emerge, they could well prove to be more effective and safer than current hypericin-based hypericum extracts.

The $4.3 million clinical trial funded by the US Office of

Alternative Medicine is comparing the effects of a hypericin-standardised extract, an SSRI anti-depressant (Zoltoft) and placebo on 336 patients over an eight-week period. The largest clinical trial undertaken into a herbal medicine, the results will be crucial in determining whether hypericum is accepted as an anti-depressant within the USA. It may also give useful information on hypericum's effectiveness over a longer period than the six weeks that has been the maximum length of treatment employed in previous trials. The outcome, one can anticipate, will prove favourable, though better results might be produced with a different hypericum extract.

OTHER HYPERICUM SPECIES

Many other species of hypericum are under investigation to see if they too may prove viable as medicines. Hypericin has, for example, been shown by one team of researchers to be present in approximately 60 per cent of the 280 hypericum species surveyed.[16] Many species have been used in traditional medicine, and at least eleven, including St John's wort, have been used within traditional Chinese medicine.[17] A brief list of some species that are being, or have been, researched for their medicinal use includes:

H. andrecynanum—has distinct antibacterial activity *in vitro*.
H. calycinum (Rose of Sharon)—a common garden plant, it has anti-depressant activity, though it does not contain hypericin.
H. caprifolium—appears to have appetite-suppressant activity.
H. drummondii—contains constituents with potent antibiotic activity *in vitro*.
H. japonicum—Chinese research suggests that this species has potential liver protective activity, and has demonstrated anti-tumour activity. Used in China for wounds, colds and jaundice; traditionally used in the Philippines to alleviate toothache.[17]
H. scabrum—in Turkish research has been shown to have an anti-ulcer activity.

CHAPTER 10

Conclusion

Better the reward of its virtues
Than a herd of white cattle
of St John's wort, from a Gaelic poem
recorded in 1900 by Alexander Carmichael

After a long tour of humanity's inter-relationship with St John's wort—as medicine, cosmetic, talisman and wild plant, it is clear that this is no ordinary herb. Flowering at high summer, catching the sunlight in its yellow-gold flowers, hypericum does indeed, as Paracelsus claimed, have 'the strength to chase [away] the ghosts of nature, also worms, and wounds and bone fractures . . . and all downheartedness'.[1]

Its range of activity as a medicine, although still poorly understood, is wide; and its role as an anti-depressant is simply the most validated aspect of this overall therapeutic activity. Perhaps this is the most extraordinary thing—that it acts on many different physiological and mental processes *at one and the same time.* Its wide-ranging effects on the central nervous system; its antimicrobial and immune-stimulant activity; its ability to control inflammation and to heal wounds—quite how each of these specific actions interconnects to produce this *overall* effect is very difficult to say, for the biological effects of herbal medicines are far more readily detectable than their mechanisms of action.[2]

Nevertheless, one can speculate that hypericum works to *normalise* mental and physiological function. Exerting many subtle influences on nervous, endocrine and immune aspects of the organism, it supports the return of normal coordination, of balance. And, to a significant degree, it appears to work *on a continuum,* turning bodily function back towards the central point where homoeostasis, or physiological balance, can be re-established. It acts as a sedative in those who are anxious and overactive, and as a mild stimulant and tonic in those who are depressed and nervously exhausted; it improves sleep quality in those who are short of sleep, as well as in those who are sleeping excessively. In some contexts it stimulates immune function—for example in viral infection—while in others it suppresses it, as in chronic inflammatory states. It stimulates repair of wounds, of damaged cells, but acts to prevent the development of dysfunctional, cancerous cells.

Taking this normalising activity one step further, it is tempting to see hypericum as having an over-arching *protective* role,[3] running all the way through from its traditional usage to protect against evil (something that garlic, another equally impressive plant medicine, was also thought to do) to its apparent ability to protect the liver from damage by infection or toxins.

Throughout this book hypericin has been described as aiding fraught and dispirited emotional states. It is a plant that seems to offer a protective cloak against the cruel winds that life whips up around us, not so much by dulling pain or blocking the sense of exposure, as by enabling us to recover sufficient self-esteem and vitality to be able to find a way forward. Ultimately, this is what makes hypericum unique: effectiveness in relieving depression and lowered emotional vitality with a minimal disturbance of normal physiological and mental function.

There is still much more to be understood about how the herb, and different extracts of it, can best be used to relieve depression. In particular, the question of whether it is effective in severe depression needs to be answered. If hypericum were to prove useful in depression regardless of its severity, it would indeed be a remarkable plant, potentially able to save thousands of people from death at their own hands. Though synthetic anti-depressants are effective in relieving severe depression, their unpleasant side-effects quite often lead to people discontinuing treatment. Suicide attempts with synthetic anti-depressants are thought to amount to 30.1 deaths per million prescriptions.[4]

CONCLUSION

The one major trial so far to test hypericum's use in severe depression produced positive results, leading the researchers to state that 'severely depressed patients can be treated' with hypericum extract. In this randomised, double-blind clinical trial, patients were given either a high dose of hypericum (1,800mg rather than the normal 900mg a day) or 150mg a day of the 'tricyclic' imipramime.[5] Imipramine achieved a slightly better rating than hypericum for its effectiveness as an anti-depressant, but caused nearly double the number of side-effects: 23 per cent of those taking the hypericum extract experienced adverse effects—mostly gastric symptoms, restlessness and dizziness; while 41 per cent of the imipramine group experienced side-effects—mostly dry mouth, gastric symptoms, tiredness and sweating. This is a promising outcome, indicating that even at double the standard dose hypericum is well tolerated.

Finally, then, one does not have to agree with Paracelsus that St John's wort is a universal medicine 'beyond mankind's creation' to recognise that there is still much to discover about this humble plant's potential as a medicine.

Useful Addresses

International links—the Internet
There is a vast amount of information on St John's wort on the Internet. The best starting point is a website dedicated to the herb and its use in depression:
http://www.hypericum.com
It provides a wealth of useful information on the herb, including products available, and links to other sites.

For a look at much of the scientific research on the herb the US National Library of Medicine MEDLINE database is free and impossible to beat, giving abstracts (summaries) of many recent research papers (on hypericum, etc.) published around the world:
http://www.nlm.nih.gov

The homepage of the American Botanical Council has a wealth of information on 'herbs and phytomedicinals', including St John's wort. It has links to many other useful sites: http://www.herbalgram.org

You can even take a 'walk' through the virtual herb garden at the University of Washington. Hypericum can be found at:
http://www.nnlm.nlm.nih.gov./pnr/uwmhg/h-perf.html

For depression-related websites, and for self-treatment and information relevant to patients, Health World Online at: http://www.healthy.net is excellent.

There are numerous newsgroups on depression, seasonal affective disorder, etc.

The United Kingdom
For all those interested in herbal medicine:
The Herb Society, Deddington Hill Farm, Warmington, Banbury OX17 1XB.

For a list of qualified medical herbalists:
National Institute of Medical Herbalists, 56 Longbrook Street, Exeter EX4 6AH.

For manufacturers of herbal medicines:
British Herbal Medicine Association, Sun House, Church Street, Stroud GL5 1JL.

Mail order suppliers of herbal medicines:
Napier & Sons, 148 Dunbarton Road, Edinburgh EH 1HZ
and at 1 Byres Road, Glasgow GL11 6XE.

Neal's Yard Remedies, 15 Neal's Yard, Covent Garden, London WC2 9DP
and at Chelsea Farmers Market, Sydney Street, London SW3 6NR.

The USA
Herbal Medicine Associations:
American Association of Naturopathic Physicians, 2366 Eastlake Avenue East, Ste. 322, Seattle, WA 98102.

American Herb Association, PO Box 1673, Nevada City, CA 95959.

American Herbalists Guild, PO Box 1683, Soquel, CA 95073.

Association of Natural Medicine Pharmacists, 8369 Champs De Elysses, Forestville, CA 95436.

Eclectic Institute, 11231 SE Market Street, Portland, OR 97216.

Herb Research Foundation, 1007 Pearl Street, Ste. 200, Boulder, CO 80302.

Suppliers of Herbal Medicines:
Ethical Nutrients, 21020 N. Rand Road, #AB, Lake Zurich, IL 60074-3942.

Gaia Herbs, 62 Old Littleton Road, Harvard, MA 01451.

Herb-Pharm, 347 East Fork Road, Williams, OR 97544.

Herbs Etc., 1340 Rufina Circle, Santa Fe, NM 87501.

Kiehls Pharmacy, 109 Third Avenue, New York, NY 10009.

Nature's Way Products Inc., 10 Mountain Springs Parkway, PO Box 2233, Springville, UT 84663.

Planetary Formulas, PO Box 533, Soquel, CA 95073.

Canada
Herbal Medicine Associations:
Canadian Association of Herbal Practitioners, 921, 17th Avenue Southwest, Calgary, Alta., T2T OA4.

Ontario Herbalists Association, 11 Winthrop Place, Stoney Creek, Ont. L8G 3M3.

Suppliers of Herbal Medicines:
Gaia Garden Herbal Apothecary (and mail order), 2672 West Broadway, Vancouver BC, V6K 2G3.

Herboristerie Desjardins Inc., 3383 St Catherine Street East, Montreal, Que., H1W 2C5.

International Herbs Co., 31 St Andrews, Toronto, Ont., M5T 1K7.

In Australia

Herbal Medicine Association:
National Herbalists Association of Australia, Suite 305, 3 Smail Street, Broadway, NSW 2007.

Suppliers of Herbal Medicines:
MediHerb Pty Ltd., 124 McEvoy St, Warwick, QLD 4370.

Southern Cross Herbals (and mail order), 66 William Street, Gosford, NSW 2250.

References

Chapter 1   Hypericum—a Modern Medicine?

1   Sir Cyril Chantler, quoted in Bad Medicine, *The Guardian*, G2, 22 October 1998.

2   Bloomfield, H. (1996). *Hypericum and Depression*, Prelude.

3.   Grunwald, J. (1995). The European phytomedicines market, *HerbalGram*, September.

4.   MacLennan, A. H. *et al.* (1996). Prevalence and cost of alternative medicine in Australia, *The Lancet*, 347:569–73.

5.   German Kommision E monograph (1984). B Anz no. 228, 5 December.

6   Hoffman, J. and Kuell, E. (1979). Anti-depressant treatment with hypericin, *Z. allg. Med.*, 55:776–82.

7   Prozac *The Guardian*, 4 February 1994.

8   Cott, J. and Fugh-Berman, A. (1998). Is St John's Wort (*Hypericum perforatum*) an effective anti-depressant?, *J. Nerv. Men. Dis.*, 186;8:500–1.

9   Houghton, P. (1996). Letter to *BMJ*, 313:1204–5.

10   National Institute of Mental Health (USA) website http://www.nimh.gov

11   Bone, K. (1996). *Clinical Applications of Ayurvedic and Chinese Herbs*, Phytotherapy Press, Queensland.

12   Nahrstedt, A. and Butterweck, V. (1997). Biologically active and other chemical constituents of *Hypericum perforatum*, *Pharmacopsych*, 30:S129–34.

13   American Herbal Pharmacopoeia—St John's Wort Monograph (1997).

14   Lavie, G. *et al.* (1995). The chemical and biological properties of hypericin—a compound with a broad spectrum of biological activities, *Med. Res. Rev.*, 15;2:111–19.

15   Erdelmeier, C. (1998). Hyperforin, possibly the major non-nitrogenous secondary metabolite of *Hypericum perforatum* L, *Pharmacopsych.*, 31:S2–6.

16   Bhattacharaya, S. *et al.* (1998). Activity profiles of ten hyperforin-containing Hypericum extracts in behavioural models, 31:S22–9.

17 Melzer, R. *et al.* (1991). Vasoactive properties of procyanidins from *Hypericum perforatum* L in isolated porcine coronary arteries, *Arzn. Forsch.*, 41:481–3.

18 Baureithel, K. H. *et al.* (1997). Inhibition of benzodiazepine binding in vitro by amentoflavone, a constituent of various species of Hypericum, *Pharm. Acta. Helv.*, 72(3):153–7.

19 Murch, S. *et al.* (1997). Melatonin in feverfew and other medicinal plants, *The Lancet*, 350;9091:1598–9.

20 Bojovic, D. *et al.* (1992). Fixed oil from St John's Wort seeds, *Acta Horticulturae*, 306:236–8.

21 Bombardelli, E. (1995). Hypericum perforatum, *Fitoterapia*, 64;1:43–68.

22 Takahashi, I. (1989). Hypericin and pseudohypericin specifically inhibit protein kinase C; possible relation to their antiretroviral activity, *Biochem. Biophys. Res. Comm.*, 165:1207–12.

23 Bisset, N. (ed.) (1994). *Herbal Drugs and Phytopharmaceuticals*, Medpharm.

Chapter 2   Green Medicine

1 Southwell, I. and Campbell, M. (1991). Hypericin content variation in *Hypericum perforatum* in Australia, *Phytochemistry*, 30:475–8.

2 Erdelmeier, C. (1998). Hyperforin, possibly the major non-nitrogenous secondary metabolite of *Hypericum perforatum* L., *Pharmacopsych.* 31:S2–6.

3 American Herbal Pharmacopoeia—St John's Wort Monograph (1997).

4 Fitter, R., Fitter, A. and Blamey, M. (1985). *The Wild Flowers of Britain and Northern Europe*, London: Collins.

5 Levetin, E. and McMahon, K. (1996). *Plants and Society*, Wm Brown.

6 Kordana, S. and Zalecki, R. Badania uprawowe dziurawca zwyczanjnego (*Hypericum perforatum* L), *Herba Polonica*, 42(3):144–50. Cited in *AJMH*, 8(4), 1996, p. 119.

7 Kazmierczakowa, R. and Rams, B. (1974). The effect of industrial air pollution on the lead and zinc content of some medicinal plants in the Olkusz area, *Herba Polonica*, 20;4;373–8.

8 Ozturk, Y. *et al.* (1996). Effects of *Hypericum calycinum* L extract on the central nervous system of mice, *Phytotherapy Research*, 10;8:700–2.

9 Hansel, R. *et al.* (1993). *Hagers Handbuch der Pharmazeutischen Praxis* vol. 5, Springer-Verlag. Cited in American Herbal Pharmacopoeia—St John's Wort Monograph (1997).

10   Bisset, N. (ed.) (1994). *Herbal Drugs and Phytopharmaceuticals*, Medpharm.

11   Nahrstedt, A. and Butterweck, V. (1997). Biologically active and other chemical constituents of *Hypericum perforatum*, *Pharmacopsych.*, 30 S129–34.

12   Buter, B. *et al.* (1998). Significance of genetic and environmental aspects in the field cultivation of *Hypericum perforatum*, *Planta Med.*, 64;5:431–7.

Chapter 3   Hypericum—Herbal Anti-depressant

1   Linde, K. *et al.* (1996). St John's wort for depression—an overview and meta-analysis of randomised clinical trials, *BMJ* 313:253–8.

2   Laakmann, G. *et al.* (1998). St John's wort in mild to moderate depression: the relevance of hyperforin for clinical efficacy, *Pharmacopsych.*, 31:S54–9.

3   Soranus of Ephesus, cited in Jackson, S. (1986). *Melancholia and Depression*, Yale University Press.

4   American Holistic Medical Association, cited in Green, S. (1998). The heart of healing, *Positive Health*, 34:9–12.

5   National Institute of Mental Health (USA) website http://www.nimh.gov

6   Judd, F. K. and Norman, T. R. (1990). Current treatment concepts in depression, *Aust. Fam. Physician*, 19(9):1347–54.

7   Klerman, G. L. and Weissman, M. M. (1989). Increasing rates of depression, *JAMA*, 261:2229; and Judd, L. (1995). Mood disorders in the general population represent an important and worldwide public health problem, *Int. Clin. Psychopharmacol.*, 10 (Suppl.4), 5–10.

8   American Herbal Pharmacopoeia—St John's Wort Monograph (1997).

9   Schulz, V. *et al.* (1997). Clinical trials with Phytopsychopharmacological agents, *Phytomedicine*, 4;4:379–87.

10   Mostly in the Mind, *New Scientist*, 11 July 1998.

11   European Scientific Cooperative for Phytotherapy (1996). *Hyperici Florae*, ESCOP Monograph.

12   Woelk, H. *et al.* (1994). Benefits and risks of the hypericin extract LI160: a drug monitoring study with 3250 patients, *J. Ger. Psychiat. Neurol.*. 7:S34–8.

13   Wheatley, D. (1997). LI160, An extract of St John's Wort, versus amitriptyline in mildly to moderately depressed outpatients—a controlled 6-week clinical trial, *Pharmacopsych.*, 30:S77–80.

14   Vorbach, E. (1997). Efficacy and tolerability of St John's Wort

REFERENCES

extract LI160 versus imipramine in patients with severe depression, *Pharmacopsych*, 30:81–5.

15 Watkins, A. (ed.) (1997). *Mind Body Medicine*, Churchill Livingstone.

16 Smith, R. (1991). The macrophage theory of depression, *Medical Hypotheses*, 35:298–306.

17 Petty, F. (1995). Benzodiazepines as anti-depressants: does GABA play a role in depression?, *Biol. Psychiatry*, 38:578–91.

18 Kellner, M. *et al.* (1997). Corticotropin-Releasing Hormone inhibits melatonin secretion in healthy volunteers—a potential link to low-melatonin syndrome in depression?, *Neuroendocrinol*, 65:284–90.

19 Bombardelli, E. (1995). Hypericum perforatum, *Fitoterapia*, 64;1:43–68.

20 Suzuki, O. (1984). Inhibition of monoamine oxidase by hypericin, *Planta Medica*, 50:272–4.

21 Bladt, S. and Wagner, H. (1994). Inhibition of MAO by Fractions and Constituents of Hypericum Extract, *J. Ger. Psych. Neurol.*, 7(suppl 1:S57–9).

22 Demisch, L. *et al.* (1989). Identification of MAO-type-A inhibitors in *Hypericum perforatum* L. (Hyperforat), *Pharmacopsych.*, 22:194.

23 Sparenberg, B. *et al.* (1993). Investigations of the anti-depressive effects of St John's Wort, *Pharm. Ztg. Wiss.*, 6:50–4.

24 Muller, W. *et al.* (1997). Effects of Hypericum extract (LI 160) in biochemical models of anti-depressant activity, *Pharmacopsych.*, 30:102–7.

25 Perovic, S. and Muller, W. (1995). Pharmacological Profile of Hypericum Extract, *Arzn. Forsch.*, 45(11), 11, 1145–8.

26 Cott, J. (1997). In vitro receptor binding and enzyme inhibition by Hypericum perforatum extract, *Pharmacopsych.*, 30:S108–12.

27 Baureithel, K. H. (1997). Inhibition of benzodiazepine binding in vitro by amentoflavone, a constituent of various species of Hypericum, *Pharm. Acta Helv.*, 72(3):153–7.

28 Chatterjee, S. *et al.* (1998). Anti-depressant activity of Hypericum Perforatum and Hyperforin: the Neglected Possibility, 31:S7–15.

29 Muller, W. *et al.* (1998). Hyperforin represents the neurotransmitter reuptake inhibiting constituent of Hypericum extract, *Pharmacopsych.*, 31:S16–31.

30 Thiele, B. *et al.* (1994). Modulation of cytokine expression by Hypericum extract, *J. Ger. Psych. Neur.*, 7:S60–2.

31 Simmen, U. *et al.*, (1998). Hypericum perforatum inhibits the binding of mu- and kappa-opioid receptor expressed with the Semliki Forest virus system, *Pharm. Acta Helv.*, 73(1):53–6.

32 Murch, S. *et al.* (1997). Melatonin in feverfew and other medicinal plants *The Lancet*, 350;9091:1598–9.

33 Martinez, B. *et al.* (1994). Hypericum in the treatment of seasonal affective disorder, *J. Ger. Psych. Neur.*, 7:S29–33.

34 Nash, R. (1996). The serotonin connection, *J. Orthomol. Med.*, 11;1:37–43.

35 Kasper, S. (1997). Treatment of Seasonal Affective Disorder (SAD) with Hypericum extract, *Pharmacopsych.*, 30:S89–93.

36 Nathan, P. (1988). *The Nervous System*, London: Whurr.

37 Panijel, M. (1985). *Therapiewoche*, 41:4659.

38 Bone, K. (1995). *MediHerb Professional Newsletter* 45, reporting Kugler, J. *et al.* (1990). *ZFA*, 66;21.

39 Bone, K. (1995). *MediHerb Professional Newsletter* 45, reporting Schwarz, I. and Vorberg, G. (1987). Psychotonin M, *Interner Forschungsbericht*.

40 Bhattacharya, S. *et al.* (1998). Two hyperforin-containing Hypericum extracts, *Pharmacopsych.*, 31:S22–9.

41 Hussner, W. *et al.* (1994). Hypericum treatment of mild depression with somatic symptoms, *J. Ger. Psych. Neur.*, 7;S12–14.

42 Schulz, H. and Jobert, M. (1994). Effects of Hypericum extract on the sleep EEG of older volunteers, *J. Ger. Psych. Neur.*, 7;S39–43.

43 Mills, S. (1991). *Out of the Earth—the essential book of herbal medicine*, Viking Arkana.

44 Krylov, A. and Ibatov, A. (1993). The use of an infusion of St John's Wort in the combined treatment of alcoholics with peptic ulcer and chronic gastritis, *Lik Sprava*, 2–3:146–8.

45 St John's Wort for alcoholism?, *Munc. Med. Woch.* (1996), 138/5 (54).

46 Rasmussen, P. (1997). A role for phytotherapy in the treatment of benzodiazepine and opiate withdrawal, *The Modern Phytotherapist*, 3(3):1–11.

Chapter 4   Hypericum and Viral Infection

1 Bombardelli, E. (1995). Hypericum perforatum, *Fitoterapia*, 64;1:43–68.

2 Takahashi, I. (1989). Hypericin and pseudohypericin specifically inhibit protein kinase C; possible relation to their antiretroviral activity, *Biochem. Biophys. Res. Comm.*, 165:1207–12.

3 Lavie, G. *et al.* (1995). The chemical and biological properties of hypericin—a compound with a broad spectrum of biological activities, *Med. Res. Rev.*, 15;2:111–19.

4 Petrich, J. *et al.* (1997). *J. Amer. Chem. Soc.*

5   Steinbeck-Klose, A. and Wernet, P. (1993). Successful long term treatment over 40 months of HIV-patients with intravenous Hypericin, *Int. Conf. AIDS* (June 6–11), 9(1):470 (abstract no. PO-B26-2012).

6   James, J. (1989). *AIDS Treatment News* 74, San Francisco, cited in Bone, K. (1995). Hypericum, new uses for an old wort, *MediHerb Newsletter*, 44–6.

7   Cooper, W. and James, J. (1990). *Int. Conf. AIDS*, 6:369, cited in Bone, K. (1995). *op. cit.*

8   Vonsover, A. *et al.* (1996). HIV-1 virus load in the serum of AIDS patients undergoing long term therapy with hypericin, *Int. Conf. AIDS* (Jul 7–12), 11(1):120 (abstract no.Mo.B.1377).

9   Mills, S. (1991). *Out of the Earth: the essential book of herbal medicine*, Viking Arkana.

10 Priest, A. and Priest, L. (1982). *Herbal Medication*, London: Fowler.

11 Soldan, S. *et al.* (1997). Association of Human Herpes Virus-6 (HHV-6) with Multiple Sclerosis: Increased IgM Response to HHV-6 Early Antigen and Detection of Serum HHV-6 DNA, *Nature Medicine*, 3;12:1394–7.

12 Li, Q. *et al.* (1992). Protective effects of Hypericum japonicum Thunb. against acetaminophen hepatoxicity in mice, *Chin. Pharm. J. Zhon Yao Zaz*, 27:472–4.

13 Ozturk, Y. (1992). Hepatoprotective activity of Hypericum perforatum L alcoholic extract in Rodents, *Phytotherapy Research*, 6:44–6.

14 Kenner, D. and Requena, Y. (1996). *Botanical Medicine: A European Professional Perspective*, Paradigm.

Chapter 5   Further Uses of Hypericum—Wound and Tissue Healer

1   Hobbs, C. (1990). *St John's Wort—ancient herbal protector*, *Pharmacy in History*, 32.

2   Font Quer, P. (1981). *Plantas Medicinales—el Dioscorides renovado*, Barcelona: Editorial Labor.

3   Culpepper, N. (1674). *The English Physician*, London.

4   American Herbal Pharmacopoeia—St John's Wort Monograph (1997), citing Saljic, J. (1975). Ointment for the treatment of burns, *Ger Offen*, 2:406–52. *Chem. Abstracts* (1975):197797h.

5   Bombardelli, E. (1995). Hypericum perforatum, *Fitoterapia*, 64;1:43–68.

6   Barbagallo, C. and Chisari, G. (1987). Antimicrobial activity of three Hypericum species, *Fitoterapia* LVIII (3) 175–7.

7   Guseinova, V. *et al.* (1992). Examining the antimicrobial properties of medicinal plant species, *Farmat-Moscow*, 41(4);21–4.

8   Khosa, R. and Bhatia, N. (1982). Antifungal effect of Hypericum perforatum L, *J. Sci. Res. Plants Med.*, (3) 49–50.

9   Watkins, A. (ed.) (1997). *Mind Body Medicine*, Churchill Livingstone.

10 Rao, S. *et al.* (1991). Calendula and Hypericum: two homoeopathic drugs promoting wound healing in rats, *Fitoterapia*, 6:508–10.

11 Fleischner, A. (1985). Plant extracts: to accelerate healing and reduce inflammation *Cosmet-Toiletries*, 100;45–58.

12 Smyshliaeva, A. V. and Kudriashov, I. B. (1992). The modification of a radiation lesion in animals with an aqueous extract of Hypericum perforatum L, (4):7–9.

13 Weiss, R. (1988). *Herbal Medicine*, Beaconsfield.

14 Krylov, A. and Ibatov, A. (1993). The use of an infusion of St John's Wort in the combined treatment of alcoholics with peptic ulcer and chronic gastritis, *Lik Sprava*, 2–3:146–8.

15 Hriscu, A. (1988). Study of gastro-protective effects of extractive fractions from Hyperici herba in experimental ulcers on rats, 36(1);43–50.

16 Omarov, M. (1979). Use of St John's Wort for the X-ray study of the large intestine. *Vestn. Rentgenol. Radio.*, 4:86–7.

17 Tram. T. (1997). Adynamic Ileus Associated with the Use of St John's Wort, *Curr. Clin. Strateg..*, 125; 16:1022–87.

18 Lavie, G. *et al.* (1995). The chemical and biological properties of hypericin—a compound with a broad spectrum of biological activities, *Med. Res. Rev.*, 15;2:111–19.

19 Panossian, A. (1996). Immunosuppressive effects of hypericin on stimulated human leucocytes, *Phytomedicine*, 3:19–28.

20 Thiele, B. *et al.* (1994). Modulation of cytokine expression by Hypericum extract, *J. Ger. Psych. Neur.*, 7:S60–2.

21 Varma, P. *et al.* (1988). *British Homoeopathic Journal*, 77;27.

22 Smith, R. (1991). The macrophage theory of depression, *Medical Hypotheses*, 35:298–306.

23 Nahrstedt, A. and Butterweck, V. (1997). Biologically active and other chemical constituents of Hypericum perforatum, *Pharmacopsych*, 30: S129–34.

24 Petrich, J. *et al.* (1997). *J. Amer. Chem. Soc.*, December.

25 Bol'shakova, I. (1998). Antioxidant properties of plant extracts, *Biofizika*, Mar;43(2):186–8.

26 Melzer, R. *et al.* (1989). Procyanidins from Hypericum perforatum: effects on isolated guinea pig hearts, *Planta Medica*, 55:655–6.

27 Melzer, R. *et al.* (1991). Vasoactive properties of procyanidins from *Hypericum perforatum* L isolated porcine coronary arteries, *Arzn. Forsch.*, 41:481–3.

28 Schmidt, U. *et al.* (1994). Efficacy of the Hawthorn (*Crataegus*) preparation LI132 in 78 patients with chronic congestive heart failure defined as NYHA functional class II, *Phytomedicine*, 1;1:17–24.

29 Czekalla, J. *et al.* (1997). The effect of Hypericum extract on cardiac conduction as seen in ECG compared to imipramine, *Psychopharm.*, 30 S86–8.

30 Hoffman, J. and Kuell, E. (1979). Anti-depressant treatment with hypericin, *Z. Allg. Med.*, 55:776–82.

Chapter 6 St John's Wort in History

1 Schultes, R. and Raffanf, R. (1990). *The Healing Forest*, Dioscorides.

2 Vickery, A. (1981). Traditional uses and folklore of Hypericum in the British Isles, *Economic Botany*, 35:289–95.

3 Grigson, G. (1996). *An Englishman's Flora*, Oxford: Helicon.

4 Hobbs, C. (1996). St John's Wort—ancient herbal protector, *Pharmacy in History*, 32.

5 Pierpoint Johnson (n.d.). *The Useful Plants of Great Britain*, published c. 1860 by R. Hardwicke.

6 Lightfood, J. (1777). *Flora Scotica*, cited in Vickery, A. (1981)., *op. cit.*

7 Paracelsus, ed. Ashner, III, pp. 628–33, quoted in Griggs, B. (1997). *New Green Medicine*, Vermilion.

8 Paracelsus, quoted in Hahn, G. (1992). Hypericum perforatum (St John's Wort)—a medicinal plant used in antiquity and still of interest today, *J. Naturop. Med.*, 3;1:94–6.

9 Payk, Th. (1994). Treatment of depression, *J. Ger. Psych. Neur.*, 7:S1–5.

10 Font Quer, P. (1981). *Plantas Medicinales—el Dioscorides renovado*, Barcelona: Editorial Labor.

11 Pliny the Elder (trs. Jones, W.) (1969). *Natural History*, Harvard University Press.

12 Thomas, K. (1973). *Religion and the Decline of Magic*, Peregrine.

13 Paracelsus, quoted in Fischer-Rizzi, S. (1996). *Medicine of the Earth*, Rudra Press.

14 Griggs, B. (1997). *New Green Medicine*, Vermilion,

15 Hahn, G. (1992). Hypericum perforatum (St John's Wort)—a medicinal plant used in antiquity and still of interest today, *J. Naturop. Med.*, 3;1:94–6.

16 Gerard, J. (1972). *The Herball or general historie of plantes*, Thorsons.

17 Culpepper, N. (1674). *The English Physician*, London.

18 Bombardelli, E. (1995). Hypericum perforatum, *Fitoterapia*, 64;1:43–68.
19 Kneipp, S. (trs. A. de F.) (1891). *My Water Cure*, Blackwood.
20 Skelton, J. (1873). *Skelton's Family Medical Adviser*, pub'd by the author, London.
21 Vermuelen, F. (1994). *The Concordant Materia Medica*, Haarlem, Netherlands: Merlijn Publishing.

Chapter 7   St John's Wort in Western Herbal Medicine

1 BHMA (1983). *British Herbal Pharmacopoeia*, British Herbal Medicine Association, Bournemouth.
2 ESCOP (1996). *Monograph: St John's Wort*, European Scientific Cooperative for Phytotherapy.
3 American Herbal Pharmacopoeia—St John's Wort Monograph (1997).
4 Felter, H. and Lloyd, J.(1983). *King's American Dispensatory*, Eclectic Medical Publications.
5 Priest, A. and Priest, L. (1982). *Herbal Medication*, London: Fowler.
6 Hoffman, J. and Kuell, E. (1979) Anti-depressant treatment with hypericin, *S. Allg. Med.*, 55:776–82.
7 Grunwald, J. (1995). The European phytomedicines market, *Herbal-Gram*, September.
8 Vogel, A. (1986). *Nature—your guide to healthy living*, Vogel, Teulen, Switzerland.
9 Leclerc, H. (1954). *Précis de Phytotherapie*, Lyon.
10 Feijao, O. (1962). *Medicine pelas plantas*, Lisbon: Progresso.
11 Font Quer, P. 1981). *Plantas Medicinales—el Dioscorides renovado* Barcelona: Editorial Labor.
12 Barbagallo, C. and Chisari, G. (1987). Antimicrobial activity of three Hypericum species, *Fitoterapia*, 58;3:175–7.
13 Boulos, L. (1983). *Medicinal Plants of North Africa*, Reference Publications.
14 Yesilada, E. (1995). Traditional medicine in Turkey. V. Folk medicine in the inner Taurus mountains, *J. Ethnopharmacol.*, 46:13–52.
15 Khosa, K. and Bhatia, N. (1982). Antifungal effect of Hypericum perforatum L, *J. Sci. Res. Plants Med.*, 3:49–50.
16 Gerhard, I. *et al.* Sixth Phytotherapy Conference, Berlin, October 1995–as reported in *MediHerb Monitor* (1996) 16, MediHerb Pty Ltd, Warwick, Qld, Australia.
17 Liske, E. *et al.* (1997). Menopause—Combination product for psycho-vegetative complaints, *TW-Gynakol.*, 10;4:172–5.

18 Corrigan, D. (1994). *Indian Medicine for the Immune System*, Amberwood.
19 Le Bars, P. *et al.* (1997). A placebo-controlled, double-blind, randomised trial of an extract of *Ginkgo biloba* for dementia, *JAMA*, 278:1327–32.
20 Panijel, M. (1985). *Therpiewoche*, 41:4659.
21 Hiller, K. and Rahlfs, V. (1995). *Forzschende Komplementarmedizin*, 2:123–32.

Chapter 8   Hypericum as a Medicine

1 ESCOP (1996). *Monograph: St John's Wort*, European Scientific Cooperative for Phytotherapy.
2 Wagner, H. and Bladt, S. (1994). Pharmaceutical quality of Hypericum extracts, *J. Ger. Psych. Neur.*, 7:S65–8.
3 American Herbal Pharmacopoeia—St John's Wort Monograph (1997).
4 Weiss, R. (1988). *Herbal Medicine*, Beaconsfield.
5 Schilcher, P. (1997). *Phytotherapy in Paediatrics*, Medpharm.
6 Maisenbacher, P. and Kovar, K. (1992). Analysis and stability of Hyperici Oleum, *Planta Medica*, 58;4:351–4.
7 News release, Good Housekeeping Institute Consumer Safety Symposium on Dietary Supplements and Herbs, New York City, 3 March 1998.
8 Linde, K. *et al.* St John's wort for depression—an overview and meta-analysis of randomised clinical trials, *BMJ*, 313:253–8.
9 Woelk, H. *et al.* (1994). Benefits and risks of the hypericin extract LI160: a drug monitoring study with 3250 patients, *J. Ger. Psych. Neur.*, 7:S34–8.
10 Bloomfield, H. (1996). *Hypericum and Depression*, Prelude.
11 Okpanyi, S. *et al.* (1990). Investigations into the genotoxicity of a standardised extract of Hypericum perforatum, *Arzneim Forsch. Drug. Res.*, 40;8:851–55.
12 For example, Tran, T. (1997). Adynamic Ileus Associated with the Use of St John's Wort, *Curr. Clin. Strateg.* 125;16:1022–87.
13 Brockmöller, J. *et al.* (1997). Hypericin and pseudohypericin: pharmacokinetics and effects on photosensitivity in humans, *Pharmacopsych.*, 30; S2:94–101.
14 Shipochliev, T. (1981). Uterotonic action of extracts from a group of medicinal plants, *Vet. Med. Nauki*, 18;4:94–8.
15 Bradley, P. (1992). *British Herbal Compendium* British Herbal Medicine Association.

Chapter 9 The Future

1   UK Prescription Pricing Authority, cited in *The Guardian*, 25 July 1998.

2   *Medical Sciences Bulletin*, Herbal medicines can reduce costs in HMO, March 1998, website http://www.pharminfo.com

3   Cott, J. (1995). NCDEU update. Natural product formulations available in Europe for psychotropic indications, *Psychopharmacol. Bull.*, 31(4):745–51.

4   Soldan, S. *et al.* (1997). Association of Human Herpes Virus-6 (HHV-6) with Multiple Sclerosis: Increased IgM Response to HHV-6 Early Antigen and Detection of Serum HHV-6 DNA, *Nature Medicine*, 3;12:1394–7.

5   Simmen, U. *et al.* (1998). Hypericum perforatum inhibits the binding of mu- and kappa-opioid receptor expressed with the Semliki Forest virus system, *Pharm. Acta Helv.*, 73(1):53–6.

6   Nash, R. (1996). The serotonin connection, *J. Orthomol. Med.*, 11;1:37–43.

7   Baumgarten, H. G. and Grozdanovic, Z. (1995). Psychopharmacology of central serotonergic system, *Pharmacopsych*, S73–9.

8   Ayuga-Tellez, C. and Rebuelta-Lizabe, M. (1988). Study of the anorexic effect from Hypericum caprifolium, *An. R. Acad. Farm.*, 45;2:320–4.

9   Hottenrot, K. *et al.* (1997). *Deutshe Zeit. Sportsmed.*, 48:22–7, cited in *MediHerb Monitor* (1998), 25:2, Queensld., Australia.

10 Lehrl, S. and Woelk, H. (1993). *Nervenheilkunde*, 12:331–8.

11 Johnson, D. *et al.* (1993). *Nervenheilkunde*, 12:328, cited in Bombardelli, E. (1995). Hypericum perforatum, *Fitoterapia*, 64;1:43–68.

12 Druffel, A. (1998). *How to Defend Yourself Against Alien Abduction*, Three Rivers Press, cited in *The Guardian* (The Editor), 24 October 1998.

13 Laakmann, *et al.* (1998). St John's Wort in mild to moderate depression: the relevance of hyperforin, *Pharmacopsych.*, 31:S:54–9.

14 Erdelmeier, C. (1998). Hyperforin, possibly the major non-nitrogenous secondary metabolite of Hypericum perforatum L, *Pharmacopsych.*, 31:S2–6.

15 Bhattacharya, S. *et al.* (1998). Two hyperforin-containing Hypericum extracts, *Pharmacopsych.*, 31:S22–9.

16 Mathis, C. and Ourisson, G. (1963). *Phytochemistry*, 2;157.

17 Duke, J. and Ayensu, E. (1985). *Medicinal Plants of China*, vol. 1, Reference Publications.

Chapter 10   Conclusion
1   Paracelsus, quoted in Fischer-Rizzi, S. (1996). *Medicine of the Earth*, Rudra Press.
2   Chatterjee, S. *et al.* (1998). Anti-depressant activity of Hypericum Perforatum and Hyperforin: the Neglected Possibility, *Pharmacopsych.*, 31:S7–15.
3   Hobbs, C. (1996). St John's Wort—ancient herbal protector, *Pharmacy in History*, 32.
4   Cited in Bloomfield, H. *et al.* (1996). *Hypericum and Depression*, Prelude.
5   Vorbach, E. (1997). Efficacy and tolerability of St John's Wort extract LI160 versus imipramine in patients with severe depression, *Pharmacopsych.*, 30:S81–5.